Copyright © 2012 Gary Patera

3rd Edition Revised January 2015

All rights reserved.

ISBN:1479244740
ISBN-13:978-1479244744

DEDICATION

This book is dedicated to my lovely and loving wife who showed tremendous courage in facing the challenges of these devastating afflictions. Her determination to get well and live life fully again led us to remarkable healing discoveries that we can now share with you. She also carried and birthed our two wonderful sons, then raised them with incredible love and diligence, and from them so far we have the gift of being blessed with a very special Granddaughter. And to my dear Mother and Father who gave me life and tried their best to instill in me strong life values.

CONTENTS

	Acknowledgments	vii
	Forward	7
1	Introduction	11
2	The Winding Ascent Back to Health	21
3	New Perspectives - A Better Path	25
4	Optional Primary Treatments	75
5	More Great Healing Tools	87
6	The List Goes On!	99
7	Putting It All Together	113
8	Going Forward	121
9	Final Thoughts	129
	Appendix A: Websites	133
	Appendix B: Books	135
	Appendix C: Products	137
	Appendix D: To Do Right Away List	139

ACKNOWLEDGMENTS

I would like to express my deepest gratitude to: My wife for her incredible fortitude that enabled her to find a way to heal. To our dear friend 'J' who guided us all the way through my wife's complete healing and beyond. To Martin L Pall, PhD for his amazing dedication to research and discovering what needs to be addressed to heal MCS.

And to all of the following who played such a significant role in helping us through our challenging journey:

Drs Sutherland and Upledger and all who helped bring CranioSacral Therapy to the world; Dr. McMakin for making Frequency Specific Microcurrent treatments available; Daniel Benor for developing WHEE: Roger Callahan for creating TFT; Dr. Stephanie for her validation, empathy and assistance; Kaaren for her great healing work and support; Chiropractic Drs. Mary, Linda and Steve for the great healing care they provided; P.T. Christine for her FSM and CranioSacral treatments; Christine A. for EMDR help; Jody for her outstanding NAET treatments; Grant for coming to our house to provide acupuncture; Lisa for coming to the house to give massage treatments; Kathy R. for her late night help; Paul and Pamm for providing a healing environment; my wife's office supervisor and staff for their great understanding and support; and all family and friends who offered their love, support and prayers for us.

A cure for one. Hope for many?

Only those who have lived with Electro-hypersensitivity (EHS) and severe Multiple Chemical Sensitivity can begin to appreciate how desperately we need to find the road to complete healing of these afflictions. Only they know what it is like to be physically and socially isolated, often unable to even then escape what is ravaging their bodies (EMF passes right through walls). My wife knows from her having been through it.

With no cure to be found for my wife in November 2010, it was only my deep seated conviction about the body's ability to heal, along with the unwavering support of an amazing friend /health coach and some divine grace that we eventually put together the essential ingredients of the 'recipe' that brought about my wife's complete healing. (*Recipe – meaning all ingredients must be used for best results)

Over a few very intense months we learned what methods were like taking an aspirin that, gratefully, helped relieve a symptom but did little or nothing to treat the cause of these afflictions. We gradually found the right blend of treatments to bring about balance to her body's biochemistry, down regulate the out of control nitric oxide cycle, clear blockages in her body's energy systems, and balance her autonomic nervous system. We also learned to work effectively with the mind/body connection that had the potential to derail her successful return to work and to resuming a fully normal life.

She returned to work in the offices of the hospital in August 2011 and has been working full time since (it is now January 2015) with no return of EMF or chemical sensitivities.

While some expense is required, the total would be far, far less than is typically spent by those with MCS, not even considering EMF sensitivity. In a 2002 study of 960 people with MCS, the average amount spent on their condition was $7000 just in the prior year. The cost of all of the 'Essentials' we would now use to heal as listed in this book could cost about one third of that ($1500-2500). There is even a list of 'Essentials on a Tight Budget' that may accomplish the same complete healing for some with substantially less expense. Everything can be done right from the home if necessary.

The biggest challenge we see is the tendency to use only a few of the 'essentials', whether by choice or because of the unfortunate inability to do all of them. I believe the 'Magic' of my wife's healing was due to addressing the NO/ONOO Cycle AND balancing the Autonomic Nervous System AND getting the cerebrospinal fluid pumping correctly AND clearing her body's energetic systems AND working with the mind/body connection AND providing a full spectrum of high quality nutrition AND enough mild detoxing of the body.

I doubt that she would be healed had we done anything short of this comprehensive healing program.

Multiple Chemical Sensitivity (MCS):

The National Institute of Environmental Health Sciences (a division of the NIH) defines MCS as a "chronic, recurring disease caused by a person's inability to tolerate an environmental chemical or class of foreign chemicals". MCS has also been described as a group of "sensitivities to extraordinarily low levels of environmental chemicals" appearing "to develop *de novo* in some individuals following acute or chronic exposure to a wide variety of environmental agents including various pesticides, solvents, drugs, and air contaminants", including those found in sick buildings.
Environmental medicine specialists claim MCS causes negative health effects in multiple organ systems, and respiratory distress, seizures, cognitive dysfunction, heart arrhythmia, nausea, headache, and fatigue can result from exposure to levels of common chemicals that are normally deemed as safe.

Prevalence of Multiple Chemical Sensitivity:
Am J Public Health. 2004 May; 94(5): 746–747.
PMCID: PMC1448331

Prevalence of Multiple Chemical Sensitivities: A Population-Based Study in the Southeastern United States
Stanley M. Caress, PhD and Anne C. Steinemann, PhD

Abstract

We examined the prevalence of multiple chemical sensitivities (MCS), a hypersensitivity to common chemical substances. We used a randomly selected sample of 1582 respondents from the Atlanta, Ga, standard metropolitan statistical area. We found that 12.6% of our sample reported the hypersensitivity and that, while the hypersensitivity is more common in women, it is experienced by both men and women of a variety of ages and educational levels. Our prevalence for MCS is similar to that (15.9%) found by the California Department of Health Services in California and suggests that the national prevalence may be similar.

Electro-hypersensitivity (EHS):

"Electromagnetic (EMF) pollution may be the most significant form of pollution human activity has produced in this century, all the more dangerous because it is invisible and insensible."

Dr. Andrew Weil, M.D., Natural Health Expert

Taken from website of Weep:
http://www.weepinitiative.org/areyou.html

Electrohypersensitivity or EHS is a physiological condition. It is characterized by neurological and immunological symptoms that noticeably flare or intensify upon, or following expose to:
- electric and magnetic fields (EMF)
- one or more of the types of electromagnetic radiation (EMR) found in the modern environment

Having Electromagnetic Field Sensitivity means experiencing recurring stress or illness when near active EMF sources or emitters of EMR. Symptoms normally diminish with distance from these sources but typically require considerable time to vanish after exposure. The World Health Organization identifies this collection of symptoms and triggers as Electro-hypersensitivity, often referred to as Electrosensitivity. It is not recognized as a medical diagnosis. However, it is accepted as a functional impairment in Sweden and the Canadian Human Rights Commission recognizes it as an environmental sensitivity and classifies it as a disability.

General description:
A unhealthy sensitivity (or sensitivities) to a particular source of electricity, for example mobile phones, computers, power lines or even minor electrical equipment. Symptoms are wide-ranging and can include skin problems, headaches, fatigue, fainting, light sensitivity, heart problems and much more. **Electrical HyperSensitivity** is a name given to those who are severely affected

EHS symptoms may include but are not limited to:
- Headache,
- eye irritation,
- nausea,
- skin rash
- facial swelling,
- weakness, fatigue, pain in joints and/or muscles,
- buzzing/ringing in ears, (tinnitus)
- stabbing pains in head
- prickling sensation in head
- sense of swelling in eardrums
- internal sense of shaking especially of extremities
- feeling nervous system 'turned on' sensation of blood racing through veins.
- skin numbness,
- abdominal pressure and pain,
- breathing difficulty
- irregular heartbeat
- paralysis

- balance problems
- body and/or muscle spasms,
- convulsions
- confusion
- depression

Adrenal stress and EMF:
Dr. Robert O Becker, author of the book Cross Currents which examines the effects of electromagnetic fields (EMF) on or bodies states that it is well known and accepted that **any unnatural exposure to EMF produces a stress response in the body.** This response is determined by measuring the levels of cortisol in the blood, which is the hormone released by the adrenal glands in response to stress. One study involving the effects of microwaves on rats with a different intent, found that chronic exposure to microwaves at levels 20 times below the 'safe' thermal levels, resulted in profound stress and ultimately caused the exhaustion of the stress response system.

MSC and EMF Sensitivity/ES/EHS connection:

A professor of oncology at Paris-Descartes University, Dr. Belpomme is President of the French Association for Research in Therapeutics Against Cancer (www.artac.info), which has shifted in the prevention from 2004. Since May 2008, his team has studied what he coined the Electromagnetic Intolerance Syndrome (SICEM in French). "I have 450 patients and see up to 20 new cases every week, including children who have headaches, impaired memory, concentration or language. We have the largest European cohort of electrosensitive patients. This is a major public health concern." *He adds that __half__ of his patients suffer from Multiple Chemical Sensitivity (MCS) and that MCS and EHS share the same brain abnormalities.*

Research from Dr. Martin Pall, PhD:
http://www.ramazzini.org/wp-content/uploads/2009/01/11.03.2013_-Martin-Pall_MCS.pdf

Forward

Hope. The essential goal of this book it is that anyone suffering from the consequences of Multiple Chemical Sensitivity and/or Electro-Hypersensitivity (affected by EMF from cell phones, computers, wireless emissions, etc.) will be able to have hope that these conditions can not only be improved, but can be cured (completely healed) and will have the knowledge of the treatment options available that we found and used which cured my wife's extreme sensitivities over 4 years ago.

I am not a doctor or healthcare professional, so nothing I present is intended to be medical advice. This book is meant to be read as an open letter to a friend in serious need of help with healing

Our hearts go out to you if your life is being impacted by this condition. We do not want you or anyone to suffer the incredible hardships of severe restrictions in almost all life's normal activities and the resulting anxieties and fears about your future, or the concerns about possible loss of having any employment and all its consequences for you and your loved ones. Just having to tell visitors to your home or co-workers that they cannot wear any cologne or perfume, or fragranced deodorant is quite challenging in itself and all the while they almost cannot help quietly thinking that you have mentally 'lost it'. *My wife experienced all of the above and nothing hurts us more now than knowing there are so many living with this suffering and who are not aware of how to get well.*

I know that there are no absolutes when it comes to healing. My hope and belief is that anyone with these conditions will greatly benefit from this information and that by using the 'essential' treatments most will be able to obtain a complete healing as well.

God Bless you and we wish you a complete and speedy recovery.

Gary and Sue

Disclaimer: This book is not intended to provide medical advice. Nothing in this book should be taken in any way as consisting of medical advice. Consult your licensed healthcare professional for any medical advice to treat any illness or symptoms. The publishers and author expressly disclaim any liability for injuries resulting from use by readers of the methods contained herein.

1. INTRODUCTION

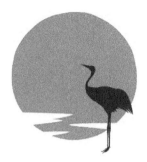

Sue's (my beautiful wife) experience:

- **Extreme Multiple Chemical Sensitivity and Electro-Hypersensitivity**
- **Housebound for 4 months to prevent exposure to chemicals and EMF**
- **Was able to resume going to public places within 6 months**
- **Completely healed of all symptoms (cured) of MCS and EHS in 9 months**
- **The treatments we used resulted in her now having excellent overall health**

While achieving a complete healing of MCS and EHS in 9 months is remarkable, it is my hope and belief that anyone suffering from these will be able to do the same in even less time with much less expense and difficulty. I am going to tell you what we would do if we started over based on all that we have learned.

Our story starts out with "What the heck happened? In what seemed like a few short weeks, our lives were turned upside down – again - just weeks after we got through the healing of my stage 4 cancer. We found ourselves scrambling to eliminate virtually all odors and electronic and electrical equipment usage in the house as my wife's Multiple Chemical Sensitivity [MCS] had resurfaced with a vengeance and was now also accompanied by a severe case of Electro-Hypersensitivity [EHS]. Her condition required her to be housebound for what turned out to be about 5 months in order to avoid any exposure to things such as cell phones, wireless emissions, fluorescent lights, electromagnetic frequencies [EMF] radiation from computers, as well as any dust, chemicals - including all colognes and perfumes, or any other mild to strong odors.

In the house, we were down to using only very dim lighting, no cell phone usage, no computer usage, no TV upstairs, no chemical or fragranced cleaners or personal care items, no microwave usage, and the washer and dryer only used one time period per week after my wife first took medication to relax her, since she could feel her body respond to the electrical frequencies from the washer and dryer. Also, she could only use a land line phone with a speaker due to her reaction to the handheld receiver and even to the use of a headset we had purchased with the hopes it would be okay for her.

While I had over 35 years of experience studying, using and being around holistic health and healing, I was not prepared for what we were now facing. However, because of a deep belief in the body's power to heal, I also had no doubt in my mind that we would eventually find what was needed to achieve a complete healing for my wife. From her perspective, she was terrified that we would not find a cure and she would never get better and only get worse. This seemed worse than dying to her and death is something she felt could very well happen from her illness.

Some background:

My wife had first experienced MCS a couple of years earlier in 2008 after exposure to an overload of VOCs (volatile organic compounds), dusts, and who knows what else when moving into an old building that had just been completely renovated on her job. It was later discovered that the fresh air vent had not been properly opened and the move had taken place during the middle of winter. Within days she began feeling dizzy by the end of the day and this reaction seemed to worsen each day. Over the first weekend, it cleared up and she felt normal. When it returned after being back to work a few days, she went to the doctor to see if they could find anything wrong. They couldn't find anything, but within a week or so we realized there was some connection with being at work. I began suspecting a reaction to exposure to VOCs and chemicals after going to the building with her to see what had actually been done there. With my background in construction I was aware of how potent the commonly used materials are, and I could see that the ventilation was a very old style system and at best would not have very good air exchange.

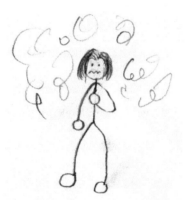

She cut back her hours to half-time at work and soon the doctors noticed a new raspy sound in her lungs. She was sent to an allergist and had numerous tests, and the final diagnosis was sick building syndrome. While this doctor was considered one of the best allergy experts in our state, he only said "we don't know much about this".

Within just a few weeks she began to work from home and we started our search for resolving what we now realized was Multiple Chemical Sensitivity. I'll never forget a ride home on a cold winter day during this time and we had to have the windows down in the car because it was the first time she experienced a major reaction to the cologne I was wearing.

While she was able to return to the workplace in a couple of months, it was in a different position altogether and a totally different building. It was quite a struggle though, and she had to come home some days when a co-worker wore cologne or was wearing something which had been treated with a strong fabric softener, and so on.

By August that year, 2008, we had found out about a treatment called NAET and went to an outstanding practitioner, who is also a Naturopath. It was a 5 ½ hour drive one way for us, but her experience and training made it worth the time and expense to make the trip. The treatments proved to be quite effective at bringing relief from the chemical sensitivities and it became easier to be in the workplace and function in life. She especially recalls finally being 'ready' for and getting the NAET treatment for formaldehyde in late November of that year because of the tremendous improvement it made for her comfort level in most everyday circumstances.

After several months of the NAET treatments and use of several homeopathic remedies, she did pretty well in most circumstances. She still could not be around things like campfires, or in a car with strong cologne or perfumes. Any stays at a hotel/motel were tricky as well and required always getting a room with a window, and one that had not recently been remodeled. We would also need to call ahead and request that they did not use strong fragrances when cleaning and so on. She remained at this fairly stable and functional level until the fall of 2010. Oddly enough, my wife's spiral downward began when she was allowed to work from home again because the area where her office was located was going to be remodeled.

I had just completed 6 months of intense chemotherapy in late June. While I had held up really well from the intensive nutritional and integrative care (I'll have a guide for cancer care soon!), we were just starting to get back to some normalcy in our lives. My wife had been a real angel and real trooper during my treatments. She was always making sure she did everything she could to help like stopping all the time at Whole Foods after work to get whatever I might want or need. She would stay awake late with me to be there ready to do whatever she could to help, then she would sleep on the loveseat while I was slept the couch, keeping one ear always open in case I got up just to be sure all was okay, then get up early and put in a full day at work. She maintained this pace and vigilance for over 7 months.

That September was when my wife started working at home. I was back at my job, working part-time from home as well. Both of us were working in kitchen with a wireless router a few feet away. She would work on a laptop at our kitchen table and I was on the desktop computer at the desk next to the table. After a few weeks she began feeling weak much of the time so she went in to see her doctor and have some blood work done. By the time of the appointment she had realized that she would feel a sense of weakness and dizziness as soon as she sat down and turned on the laptop computer to begin her work day. The doctor did not find anything and while he was polite he stated he had not heard of any problems connected with being exposed to laptop computers. Her blood work came back normal, and the doctor suspected she may have some type of viral infection that would probably clear up in a week or two.

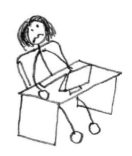

Over the next several weeks her feelings of weakness increased along with her reactions to EMF from the laptop. We took a number of steps in an attempt to mitigate her EMF exposure. We bought special stick-on discs designed to reduce the EMF for the laptop, our desktop computer and monitor, and our cell phones. I eliminated the wireless and used a standard router that I put out in the garage. Her sensitivity and response still was worsening. She started cutting way back on her hours of work, and would spend only 15-30 minutes at a time on the computer.

We had a few events that highlighted just how significant my wife's sensitivities had become. The first one occurred while we were returning home from a trip to Minnesota to see her NAET practitioner. When we stopped to get something to eat, we knew that the facility had wireless in it so my wife stayed in the car while I went inside. Even then, she could feel a reaction that was like what she would feel being in front of the laptop computer. She had been fine in the car up until then, we did not have cell phones on, and so we expected her to not have any problem. Her reaction had to be from the wireless inside the building. Remember, EMF does pass right through walls, and this was one time it was experienced firsthand.

Another defining event – and a scary one for my wife – was when she decided to listen to a message left on her cell phone, which she had not used in over a month. She set the phone down, and leaned over it to hear the message rather than holding it up to her ear. Within seconds, almost her entire body was flush red and warm and this lasted for about 20 minutes. I had read about this as a reaction that some people first experience when they develop Electro-Hypersensitivity (sensitive to EMF and other types of electrical radiation), but I had never told her about it because I did not want to alarm her or put any expectations in her subconscious. So she had no idea that this was somewhat common as a reaction to EMF from computer monitors, computers, etc. A few weeks later we had a service man here to see about getting our satellite dish moved because it was located on the roof right above our bedroom, and he stepped inside the house for a few minutes. Well, we forgot to ask him not use his cell phone in the house, and to please turn it off. He called his office to check on something and even though my wife was in another area of the house, she became flush red all over and warm to the touch again, just as she had reacted to her own cell phone a few weeks earlier. Her sensitivity to all fragrances was rapidly escalating now as well. She was now no longer able to work at all, even from home.

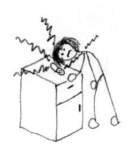

The search was in full-steam for ways to better mitigate any EMF, eliminate all fragrances, and most importantly find a cure. Complicating the situation was the fact that all exposures to EMF or chemicals made her condition worse, which we understood by her own experience and that of others with this condition, and was even further substantiated by the incredible research of Martin Pall,

PhD[Professor Emeritus of Biochemistry and Basic Medical Sciences, Washington State University and Research Director of the Tenth Paradigm Research Group]. His work confirms that additional exposure excites the already out of control nitric oxide [NO/OHNOO] cycle – like providing more oxygen to a fire. This meant that she needed to stay in a controlled environment and could no longer leave the house.

Somehow, through searching the Internet, I discovered Dr. Martin Pall's work and bought his book "Explaining Unexplained Illnesses". We also learned of his program of nutritional supplementation (protocol) which he had developed for treating MCS [NO/ONOO cycle]. I was able to find out directly from him that in the experience of physicians working with MSC patients who also have EHS, when the MCS improves the EHS gets better as well. We immediately ordered a three months' supply.

By now I was working my 4 hours at our local Community Center, because we could have no computer use in the house. We had connected with 'J', a remarkable friend who has a great deal of experience assisting friends through major health crises. Almost single handedly she managed to keep my wife on a healing path and guided us through what turned out to be an incredible maze of healing modalities while I kept

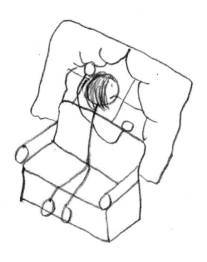

researching and finding things that contributed to what was ultimately her total cure. In all, we used about 35-40 different healing 'tools'[remember-we were learning like Edison with the light bulb filament] including herbs, vitamins and minerals, homeopathic remedies, various energy healing methods, emotional healing techniques such as EMDR, EFT and Arch Healing. We used acupuncture, Chinese herbs, massage, Network Chiropractic,

NAET, super foods, Healing Touch (chakra opening/balancing), Qigong, 'Metamorphosis', mind/body therapies, remote energy healing, art therapy, music therapy, and more. After about 4 months she got well enough to leave the house which made it possible to get the CranioSacral Therapy and Frequency Specific Micro-current treatments which finally resolved her insomnia and heart palpitations. We just could not get under control for the last several months of her healing with any of the other treatments we were using at that time. This allowed her to finally get the rest and relief from anxiety she needed to complete her healing process and resume all normal activities.

She found a great way to test the waters with normal, daily activities and contact by volunteering at our local library. This provided an excellent way for her to gain the confidence that she was in fact healed from her sensitivities. Within about 6 weeks she took the steps of getting back into the workplace by starting out working a few hours per day and increasing the amount of time over several weeks until she was back to full-time hours in September 2011, and which she has successfully maintained for over a 3 years now (as of the date of this book revision 8-27-15). In **Chapter 8** this transitional phase is discussed in more detail since it was a critical component in completing her healing journey, and involved its own unique dynamics to navigate.

***PLEASE SEE APPENDIX D** for a list of thoughts on What To Do right away for MCS and/or EMF Sensitivity!*

Our dear 'helper' friend called us pioneers in our healing journey because we saw no cures available online or in books for EHS, only avoidance was discussed. We also knew that it is rare to cure such extreme MCS and most people feel fortunate to get it to be manageable after years of effort. Our only goal was complete and total healing or cure – so I guess we were like pioneers in finding that 'cure'.

Our vantage point now enables us to see what could have been an even more effective approach. Like taking a long winding path to get to the top of the hill –we now can see very clearly the much straighter path that we had not seen from the bottom of the hill and could have taken instead. So this is my hope, our hope, that knowing what we did, what we would do with clearer vision, might provide a 'straighter path' for others to consider using to heal from their MCS and/or EHS.

Medical knowledge is increasing at a dramatic rate and thankfully the Internet makes this information much more available to us. The major prongs of her complete healing- balancing the Autonomic Nervous System, down-regulating the NO/ONOO Cycle, protection from EMFs at home and opening energetic pathways - came from newer therapies based on recent scientific research and understandings about how our bodies really function.

We feel incredibly blessed to have discovered the ground-breaking research of Dr. Martin Pall, PhD, and to have come to understand the powerful healing effects of both CranioSacral Therapy and 'Meridian' Tapping (TFT, EFT) and the significance of the benefits to the Autonomic Nervous System that they provided to her. We began using the EarthCalm Home EMF Protection unit early on and to this day we are so grateful to have found out about it. In recent months, after my wife was healed, we also discovered the ground breaking research of the phenomenal effectiveness of "Earthing" and the superior nutritional benefits of humic/fulvic and marine phytoplankton.

SEE APPENDIX D for a list of thoughts on What To Do right away for MCS and/or EMF Sensitivity!

2. THE WINDING ASCENT BACK TO HEALTH
NAVIGATING THE MAZE

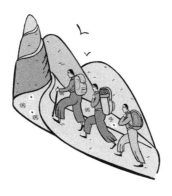

I would tell friends and family that we were using 'everything under the sun' to find the treatments that will achieve true, long lasting health (a 'cure') for my wife. That really meant that any viable, credible treatment option or mitigation tactic which we already knew about or learned along the way was given consideration and if it seemed able to address an aspect of her healing we would incorporate it. Some things were used all the way through her healing. Some were used only for a while because either they had seemed to accomplish what they could, or were intended to, or that she had reached a different stage of healing and a different need had evolved.

After her healing was complete, I listed every type of treatment that we used along the way as we were learning. I categorized them into 4 types of healing. Here are the totals Physical-24, Energetic-12, Emotional-8 (Mind/Body), and Mental-4 (Mind/Body).

While not identified as one of the categories, a spiritual component was an integral part of her healing with a wealth of prayers being said by us and our dear family and friends for both guidance and healing.

It amazes me that we used so many healing methods. We are forever grateful for the benefits received by each one and we attribute them to enabling her to make it through the crisis. A special acknowledgement goes to both the powerful group healing sessions which helped in her belief that she could get well .

SPECIAL NOTE: *We would only be using a handful of these modalities/treatments plus a few new things if we were starting over.* This is simply a 'recap' of the range of treatments and modalities that my wife used during our 'learning process'. **Please see Chapters 3 as well as the "Essentials" and "Essentials on a Tight Budget" lists in Chapter 7 for what specific treatments we would use now if starting over** based on resources available.

Phase 1:

NMT - NeuroModulation Technique [www.nmt.md.com]

NAET - Nambudripad's Allergy Elimination Technique [www.naet.com]

Detoxing baths [www.magneticclay.com]

Detoxing herbs (from N.D. - Naturopathic Physician) [www.naturopathic.org]

Detoxing w/Sonne's #7 Colloidal Bentonite [www.sonnes.com]

Flower Remedies (from N.D.- Naturopathic Physician) [www.naturopathic.org]

EMF protective discs

Q-Link EMF protective pendant

Homeopathic remedies (from N.D.- Naturopathic Physician) [www.naturopathic.org]

Energy Healing/Homeopathic [www.kosmicMatrixHealing.com]

Phase 2:

Allergy Research Group Nutritional Support Protocol – based on Martin Pall's [PhD] research [www.thetenthparadigm.org]

Dietary protocol

Earth Calm whole house EMF protective device [www.earthcalm.com]

EMF Shielding for electronic equipment

W.H.E.E. – Whole Health Easily and Effectively [www.wholistichealigresearch.com]

Hawaiian Arch Healing

Long distance energy healing [www.liferadiant.com]

PSYCH-K [www.psych-k.com]

Healing Touch [www.healingtouchinternational.org]

EMDR – Eye Movement and Desensitization and Reprocessing [www.emdr.com]

Network Chiropractic [www.associationfornetworkcare.com]

Artistic expression

Writing (typing)

Massage

Prescription medications (for anxiety, insomnia, heart palpitations)

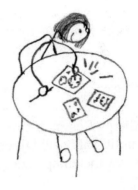

Phase 3:

Acupuncture

Chinese herbs

Classical Homeopathy

HeartMath [www.heartmath.org]

CranioSacral Therapy [www.upledger.com; www.craniosacraltherapy.org]

Frequency Specific Microcurrent [www.frequencyspecific.com]

Professional Counseling

EFT - Emotional Freedom Technique [www.emofree.com]

Music Therapy

3. NEW PERSPECTIVES –A BETTER PATH
THE TREATMENT ESSENTIALS

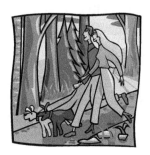

Before getting into the steps for healing I want to humbly share some perspectives I have which are based on experiences of helping others who are faced with these afflictions and the incredible challenge to heal them.

The very real financial limitations and social isolation most are facing is already overwhelming. Most often a lot of money and hard work has already been put toward following other paths for healing that have not resolved the problem. The 'magic bullet' that seemed to heal some people just did not work for them, or work well enough - even after valiant efforts and sacrifices were made. The tendency to look for the 'one or two things' that will heal them seems to remain for many we have had contact with.

While I know many have been struggling for much longer than my wife, we experienced the same things. My total obsession to find a 'cure', my perspective on the relationship between all systems of the body and its ability to heal, and the good fortune to be able to find ways to scrape together enough money to keep going were certainly key factors. Support from our very dear healing friend was huge.

Perhaps most important of all may have been my wife's and my commitment to give 100% to whatever we tried. No shortcuts, no getting loose with times to take something, no forgetting, accepting that sometimes she would feel worse before feeling better, being patient while at the same time feeling desperate. Finding what would work was critical –her life was literally at stake. How can we know if something will help unless it is done with a full committed effort?

We have worked really hard to narrow down the steps we feel are needed to heal and yet retaining what I believe is a fully comprehensive, easy to follow, and low cost healing approach which can be done all at home where hopefully the environment has been made safe from chemical toxins and EMF. It often works best to have an easy to follow daily schedule/routine so we do not forget to do the techniques(TFT meridian Tapping; Un-Switching Technique; "chi machine/or mini trampoline; Craniosacral Still Point Inducer; supplements and nutrition) which take only a few minutes but have significant accumulative benefits

Our hope is that readers will have enough confidence in what is offered here and can find the minimal resources required to fully commit to trying this approach (Chapter 7: Essentials or Essentials on a Tight Budget) for at least several months. No picking and choosing, but doing all of them. At a minimum, everything in the Essentials lists would typically be viewed as being very beneficial to overall health.

We pray for the day when we can find a way to provide the funds to enough people with MCS and EMF sensitivity that would be fully committed to follow the Essentials 100% so we can confirm that these steps will heal these afflictions for most people and let them live life fully as my wife has been doing for the past three years.

THE POWER OF THESE STEPS IS IN THE SYNERGISTIC EFFECT WHEN ALL ARE IMPLEMENTED TOGETHER

What I believe needs to be accomplished to heal:

These are the things I believe need to be done for total healing. In my view, none of these should be left out or results may fall short. *First I want to stress that I would treat any degree of sensitivity with the utmost urgency. These conditions can escalate very rapidly and the difficulty to do what needs to be done is compounded exponentially.*

1) Down regulate the NO/ONOO Cycle
2) Balance the Autonomic Nervous System
3) Clear blockages (physical, emotional) in the energetic systems
4) Correct and maintain flow of cerebrospinal fluid
5) Avoidance of toxic chemicals and EMFs (or mitigate)
6) Supply superior bio-available nutrition and enough pure water
7) Assure supply of adequate voltage (electrons) for the body
8) Correction of any significant hormonal imbalance
9) Gradual but effective detox of chemicals and heavy metals
10) Correct 'leaky gut' (may need help from Naturopath)
11) Be sure the body's Lymphatic System is draining

I would highly recommend that anyone who is very electrosensitive give serious consideration to purchasing the indoor, self- standing room/tent called Quiet Zone Retreat for what should give maximum protection from EMFs-so beneficial when beginning the healing process. Many of us live in an apartment or other multiple dwelling units and eliminating wireless and other EMF sources is not even possible. The 8ft.x 8ft. x 7 ft. high is enough to be comfortable spending hours in during the day as well as for sleeping in at night. They currently sell for around $450.

Essentials: Our 'recipe' for healing – what we used/would use now (all 'ingredients' considered essential)

1) **Allergy Research Group Nutritional Support Protocol – based on Martin Pall's [PhD] research - to help down regulate the nitric oxide [NO/ONOO] cycle**

> Please Note: The protocol developed by Dr. Pall can be difficult to take for some. If this was any concern I would try using the newer Oceans Alive 2.0 Marine Phytoplankton, available as of July 15, 2014. Not only is quality phytoplankton one of the richest sources of most nutrients we need and in a bioavailable form, but the newer version of Oceans Alive is claimed to be especially high in Superoxide Dismutase – SOD. This alone can help slow the NO/ONOO cycle by neutralizing the superoxide free radicals. Dr. Pall says therapy should target each of the three elements of that cycle, and the superoxide free radical is one of the three.
>
> Along with the Oceans Alive I would also add the flavanol **Fisetin** for down-regulating the NO/ONOO cycle. Recent research from Salk Institute of Biological Studies found that it is especially effective at reducing peroxynitrite toxicity. Peroxynitrite is another one of the three main elements that need to be reduced to down-regulate the NO/ONOO cycle. It is also is very effective at increasing the production of glutathione, considered the body's 'master antioxidant' and 'director of detoxification'.

We believe this supplement 'protocol' to be one of the most essential elements in resolving my wife's MCS and EHS. The protocol consists of 5 components- 4 are specific blends of nutrients and antioxidants and fish oil. It is available as a 'value pack' through the company Pro Health. There are additional supplements listed below which have since been recommended by Martin Pall to be added to the basic protocol.

When I found out that some research indicates over 50% of people with Electro- Hypersensitivity also suffer from Multiple Chemical Sensitivity, it was obvious to me that there was a connection. That connection was reinforced by research cited in Dr. Pall's book that indicates from measurements taken in a laboratory setting that exposure to EMF causes a 'spike' in the NO/ONOO nitric oxide cycle , just as exposure to chemicals do with a person with MCS. I also was able to contact Dr. Pall and he was able to say that in his experience, the patients of the practitioners being treated who suffer from both these conditions do find that when they have lessening of MCS symptoms they also experience a lessening of the EHS.

Dr. Pall has since conducted further research on the how EMF affects the body and his findings were published in May 2013.

From an Abstract posted by the American Academy of Environmental Medicine www.aaemconference.com/pall.html

"This now brings us to the last central issue, a probable mechanism for EHS. EHS can probably be best understood not only in terms of the properties and downstream effects of VGCC activation, but also in terms of chemical sensitivity (MCS) mechanisms, given the many similarities and substantial comorbidity between EHS and MCS. The target of the seven classes of chemicals implicated in MCS is the NMDA receptor which is activated, indirectly by these chemicals. There are many similarities between the NMDA receptors and the L-type VGCCs, also suggesting a similar mechanism for both types of sensitivity. MCS is thought to involve NMDA-mediated activation of both the NO/ONOO- cycle and also long-term potentiation (LTP) in the brain, leading to high level neural sensitization. It may be argued therefore, that EMF stimulation of L-type VGCCs in the brain may likewise activate the NO/ONOO- cycle and also LTP, leading to EHS. There are both NMDA receptors and L-type VGCCs that each also occur in many non-neural peripheral tissues, so that somewhat similar sensitivity mechanisms may occur in such peripheral tissues, as well. The proposed role of L-type VGCCs, NO and **peroxynitrite**

(ONOO-) in EHS produces testable predictions and it is important, therefore to put each of them to the test."

The protocol consists of various nutritional supplements to both down regulate the nitric oxide cycle and help the body address the negative effects of the excessive oxidation being created in the body. It includes a wide range of Anti-oxidants, long chain fatty acids, B Vitamins, brown seaweed extract, magnesium and other minerals, and essential vitamins. In Dr. Pall's book "Explaining Unexplained Illnesses", he also offers other options to consider, including curcumin, chlorella, other newer prescription medications, and so on (I have listed the additional items we used in the Summary section below). While his book is quite academic in nature, it is still invaluable for the practical information found in the Therapy section and, even more so, for understanding how thorough his research has been on the cause and treatment of MCS. Details about the protocol can be found on this website: http://mcs-america.org/index_files/MCS.htm

Dr. Pall's research is incredibly extensive. It includes clinical observation through the work being done by several doctors specializing in treating chemical sensitivities and/or other illnesses he attributes to the NO/ONOO cycle. At least one of the doctors has modified the treatments based on Dr. Pall's understanding of the nitric oxide cycle that has spun out of control after some initial 'event' and keeps itself in a self-perpetuating loop that needs to be down regulated. Some were using prescription medication along with an extensive nutritional program. Dr. Pall's suggested protocol was developed entirely on oral nutritional supplements.

This protocol was developed based on his own research and from his findings of what some doctors were already doing that was effective at this down regulation of the nitric oxide cycle, and its development was prompted by a request of one of these doctors Dr. Grace Ziem [www.chemicalinjury.net] whom he had met at a conference they were attending. She has outstanding credentials in the field and has also focused for years on treating MCS at her clinic. Dr. Ziem refers to the treatment as Neural Sensitization. Dr.

Ziem was hoping a protocol could be developed which not include synthetic pharmaceuticals based on her belief that they do not cure chemical injury (sensitivity). She also incorporated nebulized, inhaled reduced-glutathione and hydroxocobalamin (a form of Vitamin B12) in her treatment plan.

What is most amazing is that after Dr. Ziem began incorporating the protocol she and Dr. Pall had developed it in her practice, she found it to be so much more effective that she is able to see new patients at a dramatically higher rate because her current patients were getting well so much faster than before.

From "Explaining Unexplained Illnesses":

Dr. Ziem reports four distinctive observations about her patients: (after incorporating the 'agents' in the protocol)

"Patients seem to be improving at such a rapid rate that many are no longer coming in to regularly see her. She is now able to take new patients at 10 to 15 times the previous rate. In order to assess the progress of the patients who are no longer coming in, Mr. Jim S.... has contacted 30 such patients and all 30 report substantial improvements in their symptoms..."

This is amazing! When we first researched Dr. Pall's work and I saw this information in the book, then checked out Dr. Ziem's website, I was convinced we had a legitimate way to dramatically help with resolving my wife's Multiple Chemical Sensitivity, and, that it would also help resolve her Electro-hypersensitivity at the same time.

Taking the Allergy Research Group's [Dr. Pall's] protocol:

Dr. Pall makes a special effort to point out that often those with severe chemical sensitivities (actually anyone with the nitric oxide cycle out of balance) are often quite sensitive to some of the nutrients in the protocol. He has a recommended way to gradually introduce them to be sure they do not cause too much of a reaction. He stresses that it is very important to work your way up to taking everything possible, even if it is over time, to obtain the most benefit from their synergistic value.

From Dr. Pall's website: www.thetenthparadigm.org/arg.htm

"I suggest that for those intending to try all seven [*he lists the specific supplements], that you start with the first, trying it alone for three days to see if it is well tolerated, adding second for three days, and so forth. By doing this you should find if there are any products that are not well tolerated, such that they can be eliminated for the time being and perhaps be tested later with either the same or possibly lower dosage. It will take 21 days, in this way, to get to the end of the initial period, into a period where all tolerated products are being taken."

For determining specific dosages with the items in the protocol and for all supplementation, we used a type of 'muscle testing/applied kinesiology' to determine dosage for just a few days at a time and then re-checked. There are a number of websites and books where techniques are explained. These methods are used by many Chiropractors and Naturopaths, and are heartily recommended by many holistic oriented practitioners in the health and wellness field. One well known book is called "The Body Doesn't Lie" by John Diamond, M.D.

Summary:

1) We used the Allergy Research Group Nutritional Support [Dr. Pall's] protocol. As of this writing, the basic components can be purchased from Pro Health, www.prohealth.com, as Dr. Pall Products Value Pak. [*Oceans Alive Marine Phytoplankton together with Fisetin, or, Epic by Systemic Formulas are alternatives*]

2) We added more Vitamin B complex. We used a product called "Isotonix Activated B Complex" from Market America based on a close friend's lab testing that proved its effectiveness.

3) Dr. Pall also recommends brown seaweed (ecklonia cava) extract which we used. I found the best value for us was a product named Seanol which is available through Dr. Stephen Sinatra, M.D. and his company Advanced BioSolutions. This is an amazingly powerful antioxidant with an incredible ORAC score, is oil based so it can penetrate cellular walls, and its activity lasts 12 hours in the body compared to the 30 minutes or so that most water based antioxidants. I really think everyone should consider making it a part of their daily health care.

4) Dr. Pall also mentions adding selenium and we used a whole food source. One of the important things selenium does is help the body utilize Iodine. Experts say take no more than 400 mg per day.

5) We used 5-10 grams per day of a buffered Vitamin C and bioflavonoids powder.

6) My wife also used the Magnesium/Calcium product called Natural Vitality Calms, for stress and magnesium is believed to have some natural EMF protective effect acting as a natural calcium channel blocker. Transdermal magnesium oil is an excellent option; no digestive issues, simply apply on body.

6) We learned more by buying Dr. Pall's book "Explaining Unexplained Illnesses" and going to his website: www.thetenthparadigm.org/mcs09.htm

2) CranioSacral Therapy (CST) and if possible combined with Somatic Emotional Release (SER)

I believe CranioSacral Therapy was the most powerful treatment we used. It greatly assisted her healing in four primary aspects of health: Physical, Mental, Emotional, and Energetic. We have had several individuals let us know after reading my book and trying CST that found it was the 'missing link' for them in their own healing.

Here are just a few of the specific benefits:

- Promotes proper functioning of the brain and the entire nervous system through improving cerebrospinal fluid flow
- Correct cerebrospinal fluid flow gets nutrients to the brain and toxins get carried out
- Restores quality sleep – essential for health and any healing
- Dramatically reduces stress to enhance healing
- Effectively prevents or treats PTSD
- Helps balance the **Autonomic Nervous System**
- Improves immune system functioning
- *Clears 'energy cysts' (discussed further below), which I believe is essential to facilitate deep and permanent healing*

I want to add here that based on the understandings from holistic/naturopathic studies, adrenal fatigue is likely to be the cause of what allows someone to be susceptible to MSC and/or EHS. The treatments we used included addressing nutritional support of the adrenals, which of course is important, but they also included addressing underlying causations. This is why I think that CranioSacral Therapy / SER work, with its ability to efficiently eliminate what is termed as 'energy cysts' 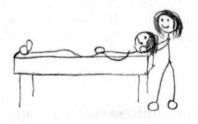 (discussed below), is one of the most effective modality at getting to the true underlying energetic disruptions which have accumulated over the years in our bodies. This helps bring about healing at the deepest levels. I think other healing modalities, such as TFT meridian tapping and acupuncture also facilitate release of energy cysts, although perhaps not as effectively.

From the John Upledger Institute website:
www.upledgerinstitute.com

What is CranioSacral Therapy?

CranioSacral Therapy (CST) is a gentle, hands-on approach that releases tensions deep in the body to relieve pain and dysfunction and improve whole-body health and performance. It was pioneered and developed by Osteopathic Physician John E. Upledger after years of clinical testing and research at Michigan State University where he served as professor of biomechanics.

Using a soft touch which is generally no greater than 5 grams – about the weight of a nickel – practitioners release restrictions in the soft tissues that surround the central nervous system. CST is increasingly used as a preventive health measure for its ability to bolster resistance to disease, and it's effective for a wide range of medical problems associated with pain and dysfunction

While I had some prior personal experience with CranioSacral therapy, it was only later in our healing path that my wife ended up trying it at a time when we were not able to resolve her insomnia and daily heart palpitations (which also contributed to the sleep difficulties because they were occurring every time she attempted to get to sleep at night).

We had tried almost everything available in natural alternatives and conventional medications. Much earlier in our healing journey she had a friend that had highly recommended that she try it for her anxiety and insomnia based on her own experience with how it helped her, but we were not able to find someone to come to the house and give the treatments during the 5 months she was essentially housebound.

Had we understood how powerful and effective the CranioSacral would turn out to be for my wife, we would have kept trying to find a practitioner willing to come to the house and gladly been willing to pay the extra for the travel time. If we could start all over, she would have gone for this therapy right from the beginning. Our experience with her cure has shown us that stress, anxiety, insomnia, and memories of trauma or stress locked in the body (cellular memory and/or 'energy cysts') were *the* primary contributing factors to the underlying cause of her MCS and EHS, the adrenal stress, and if not resolved, would also inhibit the body from getting well. I now believe that CranioSacral, especially when combined with SER is the most effective treatment for addressing these challenges and achieving overall health.

It is somewhat difficult to convey why I feel so strongly about the value of this work, but it is based not only on the powerful experience of my wife and her friend, but this belief also comes from my almost 40 years of both studying and use of many types of natural healing techniques, all the while attempting to grasp the essence of what the various methods of healing work are really about. *I hope when you read and contemplate the information below that you will also get a sense just how fundamental and all inclusive the benefits from these modalities can be.*

More from www.upledgerinstitute.com website:

CRANIOSACRAL & SOMATIC EMOTIONAL RELEASE (SER)

The origins of CranioSacral work began with research done by Dr. William Sutherland, and was brought to public awareness largely through the work of Dr. John Upledger.

It was in 1970, during a neck surgery in which he was assisting, that osteopathic physician John E. Upledger first observed the rhythmic movement of what would soon be identified as the craniosacral system. None of his colleagues nor any of the medical texts at the time could explain this discovery, however.

His curiosity piqued, Dr. Upledger began searching for the answer. He started with the research of Dr. William Sutherland, the father of cranial osteopathy. For some 20 years beginning in the early 1900s, Sutherland had explored the concept that the bones of the skull were structured to allow for movement. For decades after, this theory remained at odds with the beliefs of the scientific and medical communities. Dr. Upledger believed, however, that if Sutherland's theory of cranial movement was in fact true, this would help explain, and make feasible, the existence of the rhythm he had encountered in surgery.

It was at this point that Dr. Upledger set out to scientifically confirm the existence of cranial bone motion. From 1975 to 1983 he served as clinical researcher and Professor of Biomechanics at Michigan State University, where he supervised a team of anatomists, physiologists, biophysicists and bioengineers in research and testing. The results not only confirmed Sutherland's theory, but led to clarification of the mechanisms behind this motion — the craniosacral system. Dr. Upledger's continued work in the field ultimately resulted in his development of CranioSacral Therapy.

Dr. Sutherland's work led him to understand that he was discovering an involuntary system of "breathing" in tissues, something that was essential for the maintenance of their health. This ability is really what distinguishes a living tissue from a dead tissue. He also realized that in order for all cells to function at their optimal ability, they needed to express a rhythmic "breathing". With his extensive knowledge of anatomy and advanced sense of touch he realized that these subtle respiratory movements can be effected (palpitated) by sensitive hands. He further discovered that this respiratory motion provided a vast amount of clinical information.

He also learned that the central nervous system and the cerebrospinal fluid that bathes it, also have a rhythmic motion. As he looked deeper into where these rhythms originate, it became clear that there were no muscular functions which could be responsible for them then this motion must be produced by the body's inherent life-force itself, and he referred to this as the "Breath of Life. Perhaps this is what other cultures refer to as Parana or the Vital Force of life.

Dr. Sutherland felt that this Breath of Life was the force behind these involuntary rhythms and he realized that the cerebrospinal fluid has a significant role in the expression of and distribution of the potency of the Breath of Life. The potency 'travels' in the cerebrospinal fluid creating a tide-like motion and this motion carries this Breath of Life throughout the body. He was convinced that as long as it 'can be expressed' health will follow. If the expression gets congested or restricted, then health is compromised. The purpose of craniosacral work is to assist in maintaining theses rhythmic expressions of health.

The places of congestion of this potency are often what came to be understood by Dr. John Upledger as "Energy Cysts. Research by Dr. Upledger and biophysicist Dr. Zvi Karni led to the discovery that the body often retains the imprint of physical forces from accidents, injuries, and emotional shocks and these areas are frequently isolated in what became called an 'energy cyst'. The term Energy Cyst was suggested to Dr. Upledger by Dr. Elmer Green, Director of the Menninger Institute, when Dr. Upledger described the phenomenon they had discovered to him.

One way this occurrence is explained is the example of when we are impacted, say by a fall, the energy gets imputed into our body but does not pass through it, so it remains trapped inside the body, usually in these energy cysts. The body will learn to adapt to and work around this but complete healing of the area is impaired.

 CranioSacral therapy helps remove this congestion and 'dissolve' the cysts. However, Dr. Upledger also developed a 'sister', or adjunct treatment to CranioSacral therapy that more specifically targets energy cysts, especially those that have held their pattern for some time, which is called SomatoEmotional Release (SER) Therapy. *It would seem very likely that an energy cyst will often be the invisible, final missing piece between partial and full* recovery *of injured tissue.* The effects of energy cysts will always eventually become physical due to the disturbance of the energy frequencies and Breath of Life potencies in the area of injury.

In Dr. Upledger's work they actually could measure an energetic release from patients and this clearly implies that these cysts hold an electrical charge of some sort. This fits with previous understandings of areas of electrical frequency disturbances being stored in the body, as was postulated by Dr. Oschman, PhD.

Once my wife was well enough to go out, she was fortunate to be treated by a remarkable Physical Therapists who is a great CranioSacral Therapist. She was also able treat my wife with another excellent healing modality called Frequency Specific Microcurrent to aid with the heart palpitations, insomnia and high anxiety. Frequency Specific Microcurrent was also able to very effectively address her emotional challenges that still remained.

While her Physical Therapists had not received specific training in SER and therefore it was not considered part of her treatments, my understanding is that CranioSacral Therapy by itself will assist with some of the same somatic emotional release as SER. In fact, SER grew out of observed responses from clients receiving CST. My wife also had already done so much work on emotional release in the previous months through a variety of methods such as WHEE, EMDR, EMT - Emotional Freedom Technique, a modality called Arch Healing and several others. While these methods are all legitimate and were very helpful for managing the emotional challenges, it is now my view that they are far more difficult than necessary for the person to endure and are not as efficient as needed when we are in a crisis state and our very jobs are on the line, not when better options are available. We were using the best tools that we had knowledge of at the time. While these other techniques may be quite advanced from what was available 30 years ago, *I am convinced that CranioSacral Therapy combined with SER therapy would be far, far more effective and efficient at healing the physical, mental, emotional, and energetic systems, which are all so critical when faced with any health crisis!*

Summary:

1) We would start getting CranioSacral Therapy (CST) right away, and if possible from a practitioner also trained in Somato Emotional Release (SER). We would plan on getting at least 8

treatments. We located trained practitioners at the John Ledger Institute website: www.upledgerinstitute.com . The site will also list the amount of training the practitioner has had in CST and SER. Practitioners can also be located on the website for the Biodynamic Craniosacral Therapy Association of North America: www.craniosacraltherapy.org.

In some cases the treatments are even covered under your medical insurance, if they are provided by a licensed Physical Therapist, or Chiropractor, etc., which is not uncommon.

At the very minimum, we would use a product called a 'Still Point Inducer", developed by Dr. John Upledger, and which provides a basic level of the therapeutic effect of a CranioSacral treatment by using it 10-15 minutes per day. You simply lie down and position it under your head/neck while remaining still. It is available through various online sources for about $30 and also through the Upledger Institute, www.upledger.com .

* Note: If able to leave home, we would consider travelling long distances if needed to get CST & SER. If not we would try to find a therapist to come to the house. If we were not able to get this therapy at all, we would purchase and use the Still Point Inducer at least once per day.

2) Learn more about CranioSacral Therapy and Somato Emotional Release. The two sites above are a great start. I even found a web page for a holistic clinic in Israel that was an excellent resource for information about CST.

3) Earthing – Grounding your body electrically

Quotes from and about the book "Earthing":

"This inspired and well-researched book explains the perils we face by being disconnected from the power and energy of the Earth and its boundless storehouse of free electrons. Could much of the disease, chronic inflammation, poor sleep, and more be the result of this? A brilliant hypothesis well-grounded in science."
Nicolas Perricone, M.D., author of **Ageless Face, Ageless Mind**

"Earthing ranks right up there with the discovery of penicillin. This book is probably the most important health read of the twenty-first century."
Ann Louise Gittleman, Ph.D., C.N.S., author of: **The Fat Flush Plan**

"Wonderful book! Earthing is a return to the healing power of Nature. Scientifically based and intuitively correct, here's a simple but powerful way to restore your health on all levels."
Hyla Cass, M.D., author of: **8 Weeks To Vibrant Health**

"Earthing is a revolutionary health breakthrough that will change your life. Read the book, get grounded, and start the process of breaking the stress and illness cycle."
Martin Gallagher, M.D., D.C., author of: **Dr. Gallagher's Guide to 21st Century Medicine**

"The feedback from patients is so strong that I know predictably, as a doctor, this will change a person's life."
David Gerston, M.D., author of: **Are You Getting Enlightened Or Losing Your Mind?**

During my wife's healing she used a technique familiar to 'energy healing' workers to 'ground' herself energetically. I knew that this concept is well accepted and highly valued among those who provide or use Yoga, Reiki, Polarity Therapy and other similar modalities and that I and multitudes of others have experienced a profoundly calming effect from receiving treatments or practicing them.

While trusting in its value, I only had a vague perception about what was really being done. I knew it was something about feeling more calm and centered by 'connecting' to the earth, or, maybe just achieving a 'calming' of our energetic bodies. Since it was winter and we were inside, it consisted of connecting through the mind's visualizing a flow of energy from the feet 'to the earth' and energy coming back up from the earth and to the body.

In my ongoing studies of 'new medicine' based more on new physics and energy healing work, I came across a recently published book titled '**Earthing**" by Clinton Ober, Stephen Sinatra, M.D, Martin Zucker (listed under Resources). *I have now discovered some remarkable science regarding the measurable effects and benefits of literally being electrically grounded with the earth! Now I understand the healing benefits from the scientific explanation of 'grounding' instead of only having a vague concept.* **Earthing also protects us from EMF!**

Here is a quote from the book:

"The central theme of our book is that we draw electrical energy from our feet in the form of free electrons (italics added) fluctuating at many frequencies. These frequencies reset our biological clock and provide the body with electrical energy. The electrons themselves flow into the body, equalizing and maintaining it at the electrical potential of the Earth. Just like standard electrical equipment needs a stable ground to function well, so, too, the body needs stable grounding to also function well."

The book gives detailed explanations and scientific evidence of the profound healing effects that grounding provides the body. The 'grounding' can be done by various methods conducive not only to clinical measurements and observations, but also to use in everyday life such as sleeping on sheets that will ground us via the ground plug available through a buildings electrical system.

Specially constructed grounded mats and wrist or ankle bands can be used as well. The book includes infrared images of a number of cases of people with pain such a low back pain, knee pain, carpal tunnel, etc., where significant inflammation is present and then retook images after the individuals used grounding. The results were remarkable and measurable by the imaging. There is also a picture of a person's blood before grounding who was experiencing flu like symptoms. The cells of the blood were 'sticky' and clumped together which is considered very undesirable. After just 30 minutes or so her blood sample showed a dramatic change and the cells of the blood were flowing freely and not sticking together. It happens that this woman felt much better too.

Their work includes a clinical research of the effects of grounding: Improved Heart Rate Variability (HRV) - a measurement of the Autonomic Nervous System function, significant reduction of nighttime Cortisol production, dramatic reduction of inflammation.

Sleep was also shown to dramatically improve when grounded. *Better sleep along with a decrease in Cortisol production, would sure seem to have very positive implications for healing MCS and EHS!*

Another benefit is getting flooded with voltage (millivolts) to help our body heal. Dr. J.Tennant has determined low voltage is a major cause of most every illness, and that or bodies need adequate voltage to heal. It is also very possible that low voltage makes us more susceptible to the effects of EMFs.

One important consideration discussed by the authors is that of the detoxing effect of Earthing. Had my wife used it during her healing, she would have started out with shorter 'Earthing' sessions, increasing over time, in order to prevent taxing her kidneys and liver just as is recommended with any detox program.

Summary:

Earthing is likely to be the simplest, least expensive, and the single most effective thing that can be done to assist anyone with MCS and EHS, not to mention for general health.

For additional information: www.earthing.com

4) Electro Magnetic Frequencies (EMF) avoidance and protection

"Electromagnetic (EMF) pollution may be the most significant form of pollution human activity has produced in this century, all the more dangerous because it is invisible and insensible."

Dr. Andrew Weil, M.D., Natural Health Expert

"It points rather on the fact that electrical sensitivity will be more common in the near future. That extrapolates trend shows that a portion of electrosensitive become humans of 50% of the total population can be expected on the year 2017."

Dr. Olie Johansson

Department of Neuroscience, Karolinska Institute, Stockholm, Sweden

This is essential if you are experiencing Electro-Hypersensitivity (EHS) along with Multiple Chemical Sensitivity (MCS) as my wife did, however please consider taking these protective measures *[in addition to using the Earthing/grounding discussed above!]* even if you are not aware of having problems with EHS at this time. Logic tells me that almost anyone with MCS is being significantly challenged by the EMF exposures we all have, due to the impact EMF has by spiking the NO/ONOO - cycle in the body. Dr. Martin Pall, PhD makes brief mention of clinical laboratory evidence of this dynamic in his book, "Explaining Unexplained

Illnesses". Some wise prevention now may stop you from developing EHS and I cannot even begin to convey how much more complex the challenge becomes when dealing with both of these conditions as we know all too well by what we lived through for 6 months.

My wife's EHS escalated so quickly that we quickly found ourselves living with only dim lighting during the winter, no computer use or cell phones on in the house, no television or any other electronics used upstairs. Thankfully the television and satellite receiver could still be used downstairs in our basement. For a time, we had to use the washer and dryer only when my wife took a prescription sedative type medication. It took some time to realize that she was even being affected by one 'energy saving' type light bulb we had in a lamp in the living room, as well as the one fluorescent light we had in the house in our kitchen. Eliminating use of these was necessary.

During this time we were scrambling to learn about EHS, EMF, 'dirty electricity', etc., and how to avoid and mitigate what could not be prevented by living in a house with electricity and appliances. Early on we tried several items that may have had some protective effects, it seemed her condition was too extreme for these to provide adequate protection. *We found that eliminating or minimizing EMF exposure and/or its effects was critical to her getting well*, so we had to examine everything possible to accomplish this.

Smart Meters:

One of the fastest growing sources of EMF in our homes and lives is Smart Meters.

Utility companies around the world are replacing electric, gas and water analog meters with pulsed radiation smart meter networks, which are costing us money, privacy, and our health and safety. Smart Meters, (also called AMI, or AMR) eliminate meter reader jobs and are part of the "Smart Grid", which is an expensive wireless system installed on our homes, businesses, and in our environment that customers pay for. It's being installed without informed consent and without full disclosure of how they work, and what they can do with the personal data they collect.

We have quite a story about **Smart Meters**. It wasn't until three years after my wife's' rapid escalation of EMF Sensitivity that we found out we had had a Smart Meter for our electrical supply installed on our home. When she was working from home to avoid remodeling being done in her office at workplace, she sat very close to the electrical Smart Meter just outside our patio door. This, added to the EMF from our wireless unit close by, and the laptop she was using must have been what caused her rapid decline. Within the first few months of dealing with her new electro-hypersensitivity, **we installed an Home EMF Protection unit from EarthCalm and fortunately it must have been protecting us from the effects of the smart meter which we did not even know was there. It must have worked, she healed and is well to this day, four years later - and we still have the smart meter.** * *I don't like to push any product, but not only am I impressed with our 'subjective' results with the Earth Calm product, but the independent lab results on their product were what impressed me in the first place, and , the fact that they offer a no hassle 90 day money back guarantee shows a high level of confidence by them. Not sure any other similar products offer this.*

From EarthCalm.com:

Why Smart Meter Radiation is Dangerous

There is a great deal of independent, peer-reviewed research on the kind of electromagnetic radiation Smart Meters emit and the health issues that are correlated with it—and much of it is disturbing. One comprehensive report is the Bioinitiative Report 2012. Another report is entitled "Assessment of Radiofrequency Microwave Radiation Emissions from Smart Meters". Read about further research on smart meter dangers.

Opting Out is not the Answer

It's important to understand that it's not just the radiation from your own smart meter that's a problem. You're being impacted by the huge field of radiation coming from the whole network of smart meters in your neighborhood. A cap on your own meter—or opting out—will only give you partial relief. You need full EMF protection.

EarthCalm makes a good point about the 'opting out', however I think it may still be the most ideal option.

There is also a product called a SmartGaurd that looks effective and is simply placed over the meter with one screw to hold it on, so it is a take with type unit. We know of one person who found out she had a smart water meter in her basement and when she just covered it with aluminum foil her symptoms went away immediately. I know any wireless is very problematic.

We learned early on that we needed to eliminate our wireless router because the EMF they emit is significant. I switched to direct wiring for the two computers. While this was an excellent choice, it was only a matter of time before that was not enough and we had to eliminate the router and turn off the computer totally.

We tried special discs to go on the computers, phone, TV, printer, etc., which are designed to counter act or mitigate some of the harmful radiation. It's hard to say whether or not they really did anything. We also purchased a 'Q Link" pendant that is worn like a necklace for EMF Protection. There seems to be credible evidence to support their effectiveness, but it made no noticeable difference.

Overall, I believe the most effective device we purchased to use is the **EarthCalm "Home EMF Protection System"**. You can find out how it works along with good information and research about EMF and health issues on this website: www.earthcalm.com

The product has four levels of strength and in most case those using it need to start at level one and progress to level 2 after a 30 day period, and do the same to get to level 3 and 4 protection. The company explains that this affect is due to the detoxing that is often experienced from an immediate improvement in the functioning of your immune system when protected from the EMF. We followed this procedure and felt great relief and excitement each time my wife was able to tolerate a higher level of protection.

Another option is the Total Shield for the whole house and the Personal Harmonizer to carry with, both from Senergy Medical Group. The Total Shield is also supposed to protect from EMFs and Geopathic Stress. These are recommended by Dr. Jerry Tennant, MD, author of Voltage is Healing. ***NOTE-Synergy does NOT currently offer any money back guarantee on these.***

We can see how it is best to stay at home, in a controlled environment. For those who still need to a work or when going out there are units available from Earth Calm for a laptop, tablet, computer, or any wireless device. Using these along with a wearing one of their pendants or a band on wrist or ankle is a practical method to offer some degree of protection and helping you stay working. Again, they offer a 90 day money back guarantee for any reason, so nothing to lose trying their products.

Several EMF shielding items were incorporated to keep the television going in the basement and phase in computer use in the basement as well when my wife's condition was beginning to improve. We found a special clear plastic film that can be applied over the TV screen and when it is grounded by use of special copper tape and an alligator a clip attached to a 3 prong electrical plug that plugs in to a typical electrical outlet will shield the user form most EMF. From the same source we also obtained a special silver impregnated mesh fabric that can cover computer CPU units (the main box containing the hard drive, etc.), as well as satellite or cable receivers, DVD players, etc., and when grounded the same way as the plastic film also shields the user from most of the EMF it normally emits.

I was supposed to be working from home at the time 4 hours per day (I was coming off my own medical leave), but for a while I was going to our local Community Center with a laptop and my cell phone to work because my wife could not tolerate the computer being used at home. In part because she was feeling quite insecure during this time, she was able to be willing to see if these shielding devices would work well enough to allow me to work in the basement, in spite of her understandable trepidation about risking any set back. I put the special plastic over our computer monitor (* note – we have a LCD monitor, and they do also give off significant levels of EMF), and used the grounded mesh fabric around the CPU. I also put the mesh around the satellite receiver unit located in the basement. I purchased a Gauss Meter and tested the EMF and verified that the shielding does work very well.

I also put the plastic film and mesh on the TV and satellite receiver upstairs to prepare it for the day when my wife felt comfortable enough to have it on or watch it herself. We went without using it for about 4 months. With the shielding in place, we both think that she could have watched it at an earlier time than she did without a physical reaction, but her recollection of reacting to the EMF was quite an emotional event. It was the psychological aspect that took more time to feel prepared ready to try it again. This was true with so many aspects of her condition, as these 'exposures' caused a Post-Traumatic Stress like response for her, similar to what happens with some soldiers, who after being in war hear a loud noise and experience their body go in to in to a hyper-vigilant state even though their conscious mind knows he/she is not threatened.

The other thing we used was a phone with a speaker to avoid the EMF from the receiver on our 'regular' landline phone after my wife started responding with the same 'wooziness'/dizziness as she had first experienced from the cell phone early on. We first tried a corded headphone set with hopes it would work for her. However, the cords still carry enough EMF from the phone to the body that she still had a response when using it.

We did not have any very commonly used cordless phones in our house, but if you do please be aware that they likely expose you to EMF, especially the base unit and holding the handset/receiver to your head. Consider replacing them with corded phones or, at a minimum, make sure that the base station (with the antenna and charger) is not setting on a night stand by you. Try to move it to the other side of the room.

This brings up one final, very important thing I learned when researching EHS. Laboratory studies have determined that we are far more susceptible to harmful effects from EMF at night, when sleeping. It seems that our body's own bio-energetic field that normally protects us is at minimal strength while we sleep. This makes sense to me. So everyone should remember to be especially careful about what is near them at night – like the cordless phone base I just mentioned, or having any wireless on in the house.

The EarthCalm company has an interesting new product specifically for extra EMF protection while sleeping that is well worth consideration. It is called the Lunar Shield and is placed around the bed. Call them for suggestions, they are very helpful.

Summary:

1) Having MCS, we knew from our earlier research that EMF exposure was likely worsening the condition whether or not any response was noticeable at the time. It would seem to be wise for anyone with MCS to consider taking action to avoid any unnecessary exposure.

2) We determined that avoidance was an essential element of healing. The primary concerns for us (and most people) at home were emissions from Smart Meters, a wireless router in the house, computers and their monitors, cell phones, televisions, television satellite or cable receivers, DVD players, computer games stations, hand-held multi-media devices, fluorescent lights, energy saving bulbs, and cordless phones. We took all steps we could to shield the devices that were in use or eliminated their use altogether, or found alternative locations during the healing. I really believe that we are all better off minimizing our exposure, so we have continued to incorporate a number of these strategies as part of our long term health maintenance program.

3) We began using the "Earth Calm Scalar Home EMF Protection System" (newer units are now called Infinity) as soon as we became aware of the product. We have no connection to this company at all, but I really am not sure that we could have remained in any house with electricity being used without having this unit. Soon after we started using it my wife was again able to tolerate our use of the washing machine and dryer. I truly believe it was a key component of my wife's healing, and we feel great that we have it as continual protection from EMF for both of us.

4) A special mention about cell phones: she avoided all use while healing. We posted signs on our entry doors asking to "Please turn off your cell phones". This was based not only on information we read about but also on my wife having turned red and hot over almost her entire body two separate times as a result of exposure to cell phones early on in her EHS sensitivity. I would suggest to anyone to always use a hands-free headset so we made sure that we had one ready for my wife when she resumed the use of her cell phone after her healing.

5) It helped to learn more about EHS, EMF, dirty electricity, and other related topics. A good place to start is www.electrohypersensitivity.org. Dr. Mercola has some interesting and very credible articles on his website: www.mercola.com. It was through his site I learned of the company that makes the EMF shielding items we used. As mentioned earlier, the website of the company we bought the Earth Calm Whole House Unit from, wwwearthcalm.com also has excellent information about health concerns from EMF exposure, dirty electricity and more. The main thing I hope you remember is that while you may come across a great deal of alarming information from various sites and blogs, my wife's sensitivities were very serious-almost as bad as a they can get. Yet, even though we were 'learning on the fly' about how to treat it, she was *completely healed and symptom free* of EHS and MCS after 9 months. She had regained 90% of her healing and her ability to function normally in the world after about 6 months by using the treatments being presented in this book. I also believe we would have reduced that healing time substantially had we known everything we know now.

5) Avoidance of toxic chemicals

We felt that is was essential to avoid aggravating the MSC which can hamper healing efforts, by minimizing exposure to toxic chemicals. With my wife's condition we had to eliminate all strong fragrances, even things like essential oils or fragrant foods. Dr. Martin Pall explains in his book that a person with MCS can experience a sense of smell anywhere from 100 to 1000 times more sensitive than normal and that is what she went through. When this is coupled with the Post Traumatic Stress component, even the 'harmless' fragrances can trigger strong emotional responses. As one basic example of the mind/body connection, this stress triggers the adrenal glands to produce an extra amount of the hormone Cortisol which, in excess, is very hard on the body and will inhibit its ability to heal.

It is extremely helpful to minimize or eliminate toxic cleaning products and chemical laden 'air fresheners' used in your home by using a number of very effective non-toxic alternatives. Baking soda and vinegar can handle a remarkable amount of typical cleaning jobs. One all-purpose solution that will even work great as a toilet bowl cleaner that you can easily make is done by mixing the following common ingredients:

1 Tbs. Borax Powder
3 Tbs. white vinegar
2 Cups water
1 Tbs. dish soap (use natural type if you wish)
1-2 drops of essential oils if desired

For a great disinfectant, use the 3% Hydrogen Peroxide in a spray bottle.

We love a product from the Shaklee Company called Basic-H for general cleaning of floors, walls, windows, and we even use it in the carpet cleaning machines we rent. It does an awesome job cleaning with no chemicals, smells, or remaining residue. We also use it as a back-up dish soap, laundry soap, and even personal hand

and body soap. We also use it in a spray bottle to wash veggies and fruit. (I consider Basic-H a must have item for around the house and for camping or backpacking trips!)

For laundry, options we found were to use either one of the natural, 'green' detergents, such as the ones from Shaklee or Seventh Generation, or just use the fragrance free standard detergents that are readily available .

There is a newer product available called Bio Green Clean [www.biogreenclean.com] that sure looks worth investigating.

Of course, it makes sense to also avoid toxins from personal care items, especially from the worst offenders like hair sprays and deodorants. There are several non-toxic deodorants available at most drugstores. Hair sprays and similar products are trickier to replace with non-toxic alternatives. I know Aloe (Vera) Gel is readily available and can be used as a hair gel. Look online for other options, but I would try to do all you can to not use any standard hair spray products, even those in the pump type spray bottle.

For several months we had to use 'fragrance free' shampoo, dish and hand soaps which we found at our local Whole Foods store. These were their own "365' brand and they are great products at a reasonable price. I'm sure you can purchase them from their online store if you do not have a store where you live.

A good resource for other possible non-toxic household and personal care options can be found in the book "Less-Toxic Alternatives" by Carolyn Gorman with Marie Hyde. The Dr. Oz (TV show) website is another resource for helpful information on non-toxic cleaning methods.

If you have city water, I suggest using a filter on your shower head to help remove most of the chlorine from the water and, for baths, using a special ball type product called "Splish Splash" from Enviro Products, which quickly neutralizes chlorine in the bath water by either swishing it around in the tub. They also recommend hanging it under the spout so when running the water to fill the tub it passes through it. The cost is about $40 for the unit and the company claims it is able to treat about 200 baths so it is very economical.

6) Testing body chemistry

With any healing and attempt to achieve a state of homeostasis (The ability or tendency of an organism or cell to maintain internal equilibrium by adjusting its physiological processes) in the body, it is essential to determine any significant imbalances in body chemistry, any hormonal imbalances, malfunctioning of digestion, assimilation or elimination, or any significant nutritional deficits that might be going on. I have listed what I believe were the essential ones we used or would choose again. Some of these tests were available to us through our Chiropractor. They are also available through most Naturopathic (ND) doctors.

HORMONAL (saliva test)

We prefer using a saliva hormonal test. This type of testing is better at determining what is going on at the cellular level, not just what is in the blood. Hormonal imbalances can cause havoc on the body's functioning. If you recall, my belief is that adrenal fatigue is likely to be a primary issue related to MSC and EHS, so this test can reveal problems with the adrenals and what the best course might be to directly assist its healthy functioning. Having the test will probably save a lot of money in the long run.

BLOOD NUTRITION

If you can find a Chiropractor or Naturopath that can offer what is called a 'blood nutrition' test I think it is well worth the expense. This is not the same as blood test that you would normally get at your conventional doctor's office. However, this particular type of blood test can provide an innovative, science-guided look at your nutritional strengths and weaknesses. By identifying various blood values, significant information such as electrolyte balances, mineral level, tissue hydration and much more can be obtained. When you address these imbalances and correct them you can maximize your body's metabolic process. A live blood analysis in conjunction with this is very helpful to the practitioner assisting the patient with determining any specific nutritional deficits.

Like most with MCS of EMF sensitivity, my wife was found to have 'leaky gut' or permeability of the intestinal walls. This was resolved with a product called G.I Sustain from Metagenics through our Chiropractor. It may have resolved itself over time with an overall healthy/healing diet and after down regulating the NO/ONOO cycle, but targeting it directly up front is ideal.

THYROID

My wife did not have any known issues with her thyroid functioning. However, there are two critical aspects about the Thyroid. One, it is essential for maintaining our body's overall voltage (see Dr. Jerry Tennant's "Healing Is Voltage") and this is key for health. Low voltage may be directly related to EMF sensitivity. Two, if the Thyroid is not functioning properly and we are hypothyroid, then the Adrenal Glands have to compensate and get exhausted. We know that weak or fatigued Adrenals are usually tied very closely to having MCS.

Hypothyroidism is one of the most under diagnosed conditions and any malfunctioning can lead to a host of health consequences. One of the problems is that the standard blood work only checks for two markers of how the thyroid is performing. A much more accurate diagnosis can be made when four or five markers in the blood are measured. Even then, it takes someone with adequate knowledge and training to evaluate the results and know how to address it. Using a morning basal temperature, taken before getting out of bed for 4 or five times over two weeks or so is one of the best indicators of how well the Thyroid is functioning. It is felt that if this temperature average is below 97.6 we have low thyroid functioning (hypothyroidism).

I heard an hour long interview on the radio with a doctor (an endocrinologist) who came back out of retirement because he could no longer tolerate not being engaged in the profession when so many people are going undiagnosed that have underactive thyroids. He estimated that around 11 million people in the United States went undiagnosed, mostly due to giving too much weight to the standard test results which routinely given by the medical community. He also said that regardless of the test results, if a person manifested enough signs of the condition he would simply try treating it with medication for a while and see what changes would occur. He cited many almost miraculous turnarounds. Some people called in and said getting treatment changed their lives dramatically for the better.

Dr. David Brownstein, MD has done extensive research into thyroid and hormonal functioning. When a thyroid medication is called for he recommends Armour Thyroid (comes from a natural source, not synthetic) which not only contains T3 and T4, but it has many other factors that facilitate the conversion of T4 to T3 including calcitonin, T1, T2 and many other chemicals that we have not even identified. You can check out his website and books at: www.drbrownstein.com. A number of sites have additional information about his work. I think buying his book "Overcoming Thyroid Disorders" and "Iodine-Why We Need It-Why We Can't Live Without It" is a must for anyone.

Another excellent resource for in depth information about thyroid concerns can be found in books by Mary Shomon. More information is available at: www.thyroid-info.com

I'm convinced that everyone should have the complete tests done and have the results interpreted by someone who has a very good understanding of what those results indicate and how to address any problems. Check : stopthethyroidmadness.com for a physician. You may instead see a Chiropractor experienced in blood work and nutrition, or perhaps a Naturopathic Doctor. My preference is to treat all conditions without prescription medication if at all possible, but I have also used them when it seemed necessary. A Naturopathic Doctor may be able to make recommendations for correcting some thyroid conditions with natural remedies. Often adequate amounts of iodine/potassium iodide will correct it. Cofactors are essential for the iodine to be utilized, such as selenium, B2 100 mg and B3 500mg.

You might want to refer to one of our favorite resources for natural healing, the book "Healthy Healing" by Linda Page, a highly regarded Naturopathic Doctor. Her book is commonly found in health food stores due to its quality of content.

WHAT ABOUT HEAVY METALS AND EHS?

We feel that for the vast majority of people we more than adequately and safely address the concern about heavy metals toxicity and toxic chemicals with the Humic/Fulvic, glutathione, green drinks containing chlorophyll, detoxing clay baths, and Earthing.

While there are many practitioners, some well-known, that seem convinced that the meatal and/or chemical toxicity are the primary cause of MCS and EHS/EMF Sensitivity, and detoxing these is the magic bullet to heal.
My take is that the vast majority of the general population in modern cultures have these 'toxic' overloads' as well. It just happens that those with these conditions are the ones going to natural health practitioners and getting these tests done. So what looks like a direct link is just not so. Below is a case in point: A study done by those the Eletrosensitive Society, so any bias would certainly seem to lean toward finding a direct a connection!:

From webpage:
http://www.electrosensitivesociety.com/2010/04/03/heavy-metals-in-patients-suffering-from-electromagnetic-hypersensitivity/

HEAVY METALS IN PATIENTS SUFFERING FROM ELECTROMAGNETIC HYPERSENSITIVITY

Risks from electromagnetic devices are of considerable concern. Electrohypersensitive (EHS) persons attribute a variety of rather unspecific symptoms to the exposure to electromagnetic fields. The pathophysiology of EHS is unknown and therapy remains a challenge.

Objectives

Heavy metal load has been discussed as a potential factor in the symptomatology of EHS patients. The main objective of the study was to test the hypothesis of a link between EHS and heavy metal exposure.

Methods

We measured lead, mercury and cadmium concentrations in the blood of 132 patients (n = 42 males and n = 90 females) and 101 controls (n = 34 males and n = 67 females).

Results

Our results show that heavy metal load is of no concern in most cases of EHS but might play a role in exceptional cases.

Conclusions

The data do not support the general advice to heavy metal detoxification in EHS. *There is a link on this web page to use to read the full study*

As the article points out there certainly is likely to be exceptional cases. Of course it does not hurt anything to get tests for heavy metals or chemical toxicity. My concern is about the over focus on that issue and more importantly, the extreme and possibly unsafe detoxing measures that some promote or undertake because they believe it will be the answer. I feel so bad for those who may end up being harmed by doing so especially because it is out of desperation to be well.

7) Diet and Nutrition

It is critical to give the body what it needs to both heal and rebuild. In addition to the supplements from 'Martin Pall's protocol' and the humic/fulvic Comprehensive Wellness from Mother Earth Labs, there are some fundamental dietary guidelines we used which were a vital component to my wife's complete recovery. These are based on principals that are commonly accepted in natural health and healing circles.

AVOIDANCE

My wife avoided all processed foods, fluoride and chlorine in drinking water, white flour, sugar (she used stevia or agave), artificial coloring or preservatives, micro waved food, all meats (she is a vegetarian), and caffeine. Gluten and most dairy should probably be avoided by most especially while healing.

WATER

Adequate good water is essential to health and healing in many ways, including keeping us properly hydrated, delivering nutrients and flushing out wastes and toxins. There are many sources available to research the healing qualities of water, so please do so if you need any convincing that it is critical to good health.

We made sure the water she used was of high quality, not full of chemicals that are typically found in ordinary tap water. There are varied opinions about what type of filtration should be used, or if bottled water is really healthy or not. In sorting through the opinions about this we decided to go with an under the sink reverse osmosis system that was easy to install and cost under $200. There are also a number of grocery stores and 'big box' stores that have water available from a commercial reverse osmosis unit where you fill your own gallon jug for about 60 cents/gallon. They also sell the pre-filled gallon jugs for about 1 dollar and you can then bring these same jugs back in to refill for the lower cost.

If you have more to spend then you may want to purchase higher quality water filtering units. Some even have the ability to provide water with a specific PH setting (acidic measurement) in order to help bring about what is considered a more desirable PH level in your body. The thinking of many health experts is that most of us are too acidic as a result of the foods and drinks we take in, and that being acidic makes us more susceptible to illness.

We love to use a product called Crystal Energy [Appendix C] drops in our water and all beverages, a product that makes water wetter, improves both the delivery of nutrients by something it adds called zeta-potential, assists with the removal of toxins, and also helps balance the PH of the body.

GREEN DRINK

Another thing to add is high quality green drinks as a foundation of your everyday diet. They give essential nutrients to heal, rebuild, provide energy and flush out toxins. The health benefits are amazing in the super foods used in these drinks. There are many quality products available. * Special note: some commonly sold green drink products state on the label that they contain lead. This of course should raise concern, lead has no known value to us and is in fact very harmful. My understanding is that any product sold in the state of California needs to state this even if there are only trace amounts of lead. Some tests have been done on organic vegetables and even they have shown to have trace amounts of lead. Of course, we don't know that because they are not 'labelled' in the way that the green drinks are. We probably breathe in trace amounts of lead from city air. Personally, I am not that concerned if I have reason to believe the product has only trace amounts.

Market America also sells an outstanding green drink, Complete Greens [Appendix C].

We felt taking at least two 'recommended' servings per day throughout her healing process worked well. She also took an extra serving or so for the first few weeks to give her body an initial nutritional boost.

WHEY PROTEIN

We used a high quality *non-denatured* whey protein as the primary source of protein. It provides all the nutrients that enable the body to make **glutathione**, considered the 'Master Antioxidant' and the 'Director of Detoxification', both critical functions for healing these conditions. Most say oral glutathione supplementation is not very efficient or well absorbed. Taking about 40 grams (typically two servings) per day will help assure you meet your needs of this essential nutrient even if your appetite is minimal. This allows you to eliminate most meat from your diet to avoid both the chemicals most meat contains and eliminate the burden on your body of digesting and eliminating it. I also believe that minimal use of dairy products is healthier for us, with plain yogurt (organic preferred) being a preferred dairy based food.

If I had a problem taking whey as some have reported, then it would be important to be sure I had enough of the three amino acids that are needed to make it: cysteine, glycine, and glutamine. These would be present in the humic/fulvic product pH Balancer. SAMe and silymarin (an extract of the milk thistle plant) have been shown to boost glutathione levels.

If you use a vanilla or another more neutral flavored whey protein, you can add the green drink to it for convenience. Adding flaxseed oil is another great way to boost your intake of Omega 3's which is not only one of the nutrients in Dr. Pall's protocol but is also recommended by most natural health advisors. My wife added the flaxseed oil to her protein drinks and took fish oil capsules that had highly concentrated amounts of Omega 3 as well as a variety of other essential fatty acids (EFAs).

We just found out that the very best and sources of Omega 3, DHA and EPA is from the combination of Krill Oil and Calamarine Oil. Krill oil is able to penetrate the blood-brain barrier, while fish oil cannot. Flaxseed, chia seed, coconut oil, and olive oil are good to mix in the diet.

HUMIC/FULVIC - Nutritional Supplement

We have recently learned about the remarkable benefits of Humic and Fulvic acid, and a comprehensive nutritional product based on these from Mother Earth Labs called pH Balancer.It is now our primary nutritional supplement. Don't let the acid part concern you, humic/fulvic are actually are very, very alkalizing for the body which we know is very good thing!

This product is so good it replaces the need for most any other supplements and enhances the absorption of ones we do take. It may even replace the need for Dr. Pall's protocol, but I am not ready to bank on that yet. Taking both for a time would be my choice, then dropping Dr. Pall's protocol when significantly better. If I had to choose one of these, or could not tolerate some of Dr. Pall's protocol, I would choose the Mother Earth Labs pH Balancer and work up to three or four ounces per day instead of the standard one ounce per day 'dose'. . It is a potent detoxifier, so it is recommended to start with a small amount, maybe one quarter ounce twice a day, and gradually increase. **Special note: if you do not live in the U.S., consider purchasing the humic/fulvic capsule form of "The Gift" and/or the highly concentrated "Fulvic Liquid Mineral" from Mother Earth Labs for reduced shipping costs. They do ship overseas.**

CareyLyn Carter, a former researcher in the pharmaceutical industry, founded Mother Earth Labs to make humic/fulvic available after using it to cure her fatal and inoperable brain cancer. *For further information about her story and for extensive information and research findings about humic/fulvic acid, see: www.motherearthlabs.com*

Any healing will have the best chance a succeeding when all of our nutritional needs are met and that can be quite a challenge. Using this one product assures getting almost every essential vitamin, mineral, trace mineral (it has 74 trace minerals) and essential fatty acids we need in a cell-ready form. The fulvic acid provides a charge to our cells that allows nutrients to be delivered inside the cell and the toxins to be flushed out. Fulvic is extremely effective at removing mercury and other heavy metals from the body, even from deep inside the tissues.

Humic and fulvic are supposed to be in the plants we eat but have been depleted by as much as 80% from our soil by pesticides. Even organic farming has a hard time maintaining adequate humic and fulvic because they are used up too quickly to be replaced naturally. I imagine a hundred years ago, when all soil was organic and growing area was almost unlimited, the soil was given the opportunity to rebuild itself through the natural decay of organic materials that replaced the humic and fulvic.

I can't even begin to tell the whole story about humic and fulvic here. They are considered to be some of the most biologically active substances on earth. This a list of functions they are known to perform in the body, from CareyLyn Carter of Mother Earth Labs and reprinted in "Healing is Voltage" by Dr. Jerry Tennant:

1) Supercharge the body at the cellular level imparting life-sustaining electrical balance and life-giving energy to our cells.
2) Improves cell membrane potentials so nutrients the cell needs gets in and acidic wastes and toxins the cell doesn't need gets out and cells are healthier.
3) Stimulate immune functions and white blood cell production. The organic micro and trace minerals they carry are essential in the production of immune cells.
4) Promotes blood, cell and tissue oxygenation so oxygen is distributed throughout our bodies, metabolic reactions that rely on oxygen occur more effectively and we feel more energized.
5) Help neutralize acidity and restore pH balance which helps maintain or restore good health and prevent disease.
6) **Chelate (bind) heavy metals and other toxins and escort them out of the body.**
7) **Neutralize all classes of free radicals** (they are in a class called super-antioxidants because they neutralize more than one class) that cause extensive damage to cells and tissues.
8) Balance endocrine systems and hormone production.

9) Supports cardiovascular function-improved contractility, improved blood pressure control, and oxidative stress reduction which contribute to the prevention of cardiovascular and coronary heart disease.
10) Improves activity of nutrients received from our diets or through supplements that are part of a health maintenance or restorative program.
11) Nutrients, such as carbohydrates and proteins, are also metabolized more completely

"Humic and fulvic naturally carry with them in their structures all the vitamins, over 74 organic, ionic minerals along with elements such as phytochemicals, natural sterols, hormones, fatty acids, polyphenols, and keytones, including flavonoids, flavones, flavins, catechins, tannins, quinones, isoflavones, tocopherols, and others. All of these are vital nutrients our bodies need every day..activated into their organic, ionic forms so our cells can recognize and use them immediately..in just the right proportions..and transported into our cells right where we need them to help keep our bodies healthy and strong.

Each cell in our bodies requires a complex interaction of all the vitamins, over 74 minerals, amino acids and other elements and nutrients to function optimally. They all must be present or they don't work as well as they should."

VITAMIN D

While the list of vital tasks that Vitamin D performs in the body seems to be growing exponentially in recent years, it is also being found that most of the population in the U.S. have deficient levels of this important nutrient. This is especially true in the Northern climates where our exposure to sun is far less than those nearer the equator. As you probably know, sunlight on our skin triggers the process of our system producing its supply of Vitamin D.

It is essential to assure that we are not letting a shortage of this critical vitamin hamper our other efforts to heal and stay well. The test done through a doctor is often covered by insurance, and if not is still quite inexpensive. While a doctor may prescribe Vitamin D from the pharmacy for their patients, I am a fan of anything from a natural, whole source. It is logical that our bodies regard anything synthetic as a 'foreign substance. The Vitamin D (D3) I like is a liquid form that our chiropractor recommends, based on his own personal testing for absorption through before and after lab tests. It is called D 3 Serum, from Premier Research Labs. There is growing evidence that taking K2 with Vitamin D is best.

FOODS

Fruits and vegetables, whole grain pasta, sprouted-grain breads, brown rice, oatmeal, plain yogurt, meatless non-soy products such as quinoa burgers, nuts and nut butters, legumes, coconut and flaxseed oils and herbal teas are great choices for most. Going gluten-free is safest if there is any suspicion of an intolerance.

We tried to use organic where possible, even if it meant she ate less. I believe we get more nutritional value from half a serving of an organic fruit or vegetable compared to the non-organic because of the nutrients available in the soils from where the organic produce is grown. On top of that, we are not introducing undesirable chemicals in your body which it then has to work hard to flush out. Hunger can be satisfied with extra whole grain pasta (gluten free if needed) and healthy marinara sauce (preferably organic), sprouted grain bread, or homemade soup in order to stay with a healthy and healing diet and feel satisfied.
Consider steaming your vegetables to retain the maximum nutritional value and increase digestibility. Juicing is another excellent way to consume more vegetables. We recently started using the NutriBullet and love it! Try to get as wide a variety of colors of vegetables as you can for the various benefits each has to offer. We found yams (sweet potatoes) to be a great part of my wife's daily routine, along with homemade vegetable soup.

MAINTAINING CALORIC INTAKE

My wife struggled with excessive weight loss as she experienced reduced appetite – likely due to her insomnia, stress and depression, and some consequences from the supplements she needed to keep taking as part of the protocol. These are all pretty common with the condition so you may have a similar experience.

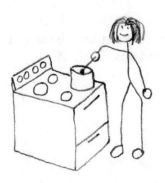

We scrambled at first looking for high caloric protein powders and any other healthy foods that her sensitive stomach could handle. Here is a listing of her typical diet that she found manageable and that held her weight loss in check:

Breakfast: Organic oatmeal with applesauce mixed in or shredded wheat with bananas
Mid -morning: Ezekiel sprouted grain raison bread with a natural non-dairy spread
Lunch: Sweet potato and homemade vegetable soup; Ezekiel bread with peanut butter
Dinner: Homemade vegetable soup: stir fry with brown rice; lentils and stewed tomatoes
Evening Snack: Plain yogurt with fruit cups (in 100% juice); banana

Daily:
- 2 servings (40 grams) of quality whey protein, usually with flaxseed oil mixed in
- 2 servings of quality green drink

Nut butters like almond or sunflower butter, which are very similar to peanut butter, are a great way to boost caloric intake and are considered healthier than peanut butter. However, natural organic peanut butter works well for most people too. Remember, if you cannot locate these nut butters in stores near you, they can be ordered online from businesses such as Vitacost.com, Whole Foods online, and others.

After she started the CranioSacral therapy, my wife's sleep and anxiety improved so much and so her appetite improved dramatically. I am hoping others will have started the therapy right away and as a result may not have to experience the same issues with lack of appetite and excessive weight loss.

Summary:

1) The goal is to meet and actually exceed your nutritional needs while not taxing the body with unwanted substances or chemicals. Basically - clean, simple, wholesome and healthy foods which will complement the supplementation of vitamins, minerals, anti-oxidants and essential oils that are already being provided by the Allergy Research Nutritional protocol [Dr. Pall's Protocol] and the Mother Earth Labs Comprehensive Wellness. There will likely be some mild, necessary detoxing of your body happening along with the healing and repair work.

2) I like to consider that lesser quantities of organic foods might be much healthier than bigger servings of non-organic. Organic fruit, vegetables, yogurt, and whole grains, are all becoming much more readily available. Nut butters such as almond, sunflower and organic peanut butter (if you are not sensitive or allergic to peanuts) are good for increasing caloric intake.

3) Find what combinations work well for you and your digestive system. If you continue having digestive problems, consider using a high quality probiotic supplement to get your digestion back in good order. My wife did. It is not uncommon for us to have issues with our intestinal flora and a good probiotic can get that straightened out. My wife also had excellent results using a Market America product called Isotonix Digestive Enzymes or Ultimate Aloe aloe vera drink [Appendix C]. Just be sure to take plenty, perhaps two or three times the recommended dosage for the first

two weeks to give a boost. As far as I know, there are no known concerns about taking these quantities.

8) Balancing the Autonomic Nervous System

The one aspect of my wife's healing that was the least understood is the role of the Autonomic Nervous System has in MCS and EMF Sensitivity. I now see that not only did it play a major role in allowing these afflictions to develop, but it also was a major factor contributing or causing the most difficult 'side effects' that she had to endure. Please note: Vitamin B , already recommended for helping down regulate the NO/ONOO Cycle, is also helpful for a healthy nervous system.

I have no doubt, she was stuck in a 'fight or flight' mode. I only wish we had known this back then and we could have corrected it almost immediately using the method described below. Without this 'Sympathetic Dominance' her healing would almost surely have progressed even more rapidly and she would have been far more comfortable during the process. Please do not underestimate how important it is to correct this!

Correct Sympathetic 'stuck – on'

The Sympathetic Nervous System is our 'fight or flight' response. Dr. Jerry Tenant in his book 'Healing is Voltage" states that almost everyone with chronic illness has this condition and he refers to it as the Bowling Ball Syndrome. The best health can come when ANS (Autonomic Nervous System) is in balance, as the Parasympathetic is responsible for most healing activities and cannot function correctly if the Sympathetic is dominant.

If you spend too much time in the sympathetic state, then physical and emotional health deteriorates and we age quickly. All the organs and systems may become affected and the body begins to break down in many areas. Symptoms, conditions, diseases and syndromes begin to develop like multiple chemical sensitivity, chronic fatigue - adrenal fatigue, insomnia, high blood pressure, circulation disorders, gastrointestinal disorders, heart disease, headaches, addiction, panic attacks, ulcers, autoimmune disorders, anxiety disorders, depression, and more.

Heart Rate Variability (HRV) is considered by many to be an excellent indicator how well the Autonomic Nervous System is functioning. It is known that our HRV is also the best single indicator of the our long term health.

There is evidence to support that stressors from chemical toxins, EMF, physical and emotional trauma, heavy metal toxicity, poor nutrition, etc. can eventually cause a condition called dysautonomia, or Autonomic Nervous System Dysfunction. This almost always will be a state of the Sympathetic stuck on and will result in a cascade of issues as systems and organs malfunction, adrenals get fatigued, and we become more susceptible to conditions like multiple chemical sensitivity and electrosensitivity. Excellent article available at: www.holistichelp.net/toxins.html

To see if we are 'Sympathetic stuck in on mode", look straight ahead and have someone see if one ear canal is lower than the other, or one shoulder lower than the other, or the face is asymmetrical. If so, we have this condition. Dr. Jerry Tennant uses a special device called a BioModulator to correct this by adding voltage to specific acupuncture points on the neck. It would be ideal to have one units for this and all the other health and healing benefits it may provide, however they do cost about $2500. While it is probably worth every penny of that, even just for this one thing, I believe I have found some low cost alternative options.

I know of two inexpensive ways we can correct this. These have worked for people I have used them on. If one of these methods does not work, then I would try the other one.

One method to try first is to use Earthing patches that may have come with the Earthing product purchased, or they can also be purchased separately. These are great to have available anyway for use with directed healing, such as near an injury or sore muscle. Place one on the right side of the neck on at the location identified as the Autonomic Reset point on each side of the neck. It is located slightly below the midway point of the distance from the bottom of the ear lobe to the shoulder, and on a line drawn straight down along the outer back edge of the ear. Hook up the grounding cord per directions, and leave hooked up for approximately 3 hours. This may need to be repeated several times until correction is obtained and it holds.

The other option is to use Life Wave 'Energy' patches [lifewave.com], applying one on each side of the neck (White patch on right side and Tan patch on left side) on the 'Autonomic Reset' point on the right side of the neck and the same location on the left side [a little beyond half way down the distance between bottom of ear lobe and shoulder, and centered on a line straight down from the outer edge of ear]. Leave on about 6 -8 hours and recheck ear lobes. If they are level, recheck them periodically (shoulders take longer to level out – about 24 hours). If not, reapply the next day, then recheck. Re-apply as needed to keep level.

Another way to check for 'Sympathetic on' and confirm the correction has been made after: if asked to stand still (relaxed)our body will not naturally sway. After correction, our body will feel like it is very gently trying to rock back and forth about 10 times per minute when standing still.

Recheck every week or so to confirm it did not revert back to being stuck on.

See Dr. Tennant's book "Voltage is Healing" for more info about Bowling Ball Syndrome, or see him demonstrate it on YouTube.

TFT - Thought Field Therapy meridian tapping

We would use TFT regularly, like several times a day. TFT has shown its ability to dramatically improve Heart Rate Variability readings, especially when it the reading is very low to begin with. As mentioned above, this improvement is regarded by many to be a clear indicator of an improvement in the balance of the Autonomic Nervous System.

We can effectively do the tapping ourselves, learning from a book ("Tapping The Healer Within") or by free downloadable instructions. Some TFT practitioners are trained to assist you over the phone. In doing so, they can provide a customized tapping sequence for you and may dramatically increase the benefits you derive from your tapping.

The best option would be to locate a TFT practitioner who is certified to work with you over the phone. She/he can give you customized tapping sequences to most effectively address your needs. Practitioners can be found all over the globe. Go to www.rogercallahan.com and use their practitioner search.

The Thought Field Therapy organization is so confident about this that it highly encourages the purchase of quality HRV measuring devices by their therapists they are training to verify this improvement to their clients. The therapists using them have consistently confirmed these results.

Excerpt from www.rogercallahan.com

Dr. Royal's Important Discovery
By Roger Callahan, PhD.

"In July, 1998, I received a phone call from a physician in Las Vegas, Nevada. Fuller Royal, MD, was calling me to report some exciting news about his use of Thought Field Therapy.

Dr. Royal is Director of a medical clinic in Las Vegas. Dr. Royal is a pioneer in exploring new treatments that may benefit his patients.

He told me that he had been giving a lecture at a Southern California college. After the lecture a student asked if he were familiar with the Callahan Techniques.

He was not, but based on what this student reported Dr. Royal called my office and requested information about Callahan Techniques Thought Field Therapy (TFT).

Dr. Royal is an excellent scientist as well as a good physician, and uses objective measures to judge the effectiveness of his various treatments.

When I arrived in Las Vegas to observe how he was using TFT with his medical patients, he introduced me to a remarkable piece of equipment that measures HEART RATE VARIABILITY. The scientific advantage of this equipment which measures heart rate variability as well as the status of the autonomic nervous system, is that it is not responsive to placebo or suggestion.

Among other things, it measures the degree of imbalance in the autonomic nervous system (ANS). When a person is under stress the ANS goes out of balance.

Dr. Royal showed me the HRV graphs of a number of patients, who he had helped dramatically with their complaining symptom with a simple TFT algorithm. The graphs showed clearly that the HRV dramatically improved in all cases tested that day. This result correlated with the patients' report that the complaining symptoms were greatly reduced or completely gone!"

You can download free tapping instructions online:
http://tfttraumarelief.com/instructions-for-tft-trauma-relief-technique/
Us this TFT tapping routine 4-5 times daily to help achieve and/or maintain a balanced ANS.

10) Lymphatic System

The often overlooked Lymphatic System – so important for good health, and maybe a **strong connection with MCS**! In his book "Healing Is Voltage" Dr. Jerry Tennant discusses how essential it is that our lymph system is draining waste proteins (cellular sewage) from our body. He explains that if it does not drain as it should then these waste proteins are everywhere and it 'drives the immune system crazy'.

From the book: "The longer your lymphatics are obstructed, the more different antibodies you make until you become allergic to almost everything. Now you are called 'chemically sensitive'." Dr. Jerry Tennant

It is also interesting to note that Linda Page, a leading Naturopath and author of Healthy Healing (a naturopathic bible!) talks about a strong connection between the functioning of the liver and a healthy lymphatic system. She also suggests that a sluggish liver is one of the first things to address when experiencing signs of MCS. So, tying the three together for us...liver, lymph, and MCS.

Dr. Tenant and many others recommend using a mini-trampoline (rebounders) as a very good way to help assure proper drainage. The lower priced ones cost $30-40 and will last for years. I would say start out slow..using it a few minutes every other day or so, and gradually increase the time to minutes or so every other day.

A 'chi-machine' is another excellent way to do this and it also has the reported benefit of helping the all-important Autonomic Nervous System as well as promoting blood circulation. While the actual chi machine are what professionals would use, we have a less expensive version called a Healthy Swinger ($100) and we believe it works well enough.

Leaky Gut

Intestinal permeability is a significant health problem and appears to be an almost universal problem with MSC and EHS/EMF Sensitivity. Dr. Martin Pall's work discusses how the out of control NO/ONOO Cycle is a primary cause of this. Getting that under control, down-regulating the NO/ONOO cycle as described above, will go a long way to correct it especially when following a healthy diet and using pure water.

Balancing the Autonomic Nervous System will also go a long way to help this. Remember the Parasympathetic Nervous System controls digestion and if we are operating in 'Sympathetic Dominance'(stuck in fight or flight) our digestive functioning will almost certainly be impaired.

Two excellent additions for helping the gut heal are **G. I. Sustain** by Metagenics (may need to purchase through health practitioner) and a high quality Aloe Vera juice (e.g. Ultimate Aloe from Market America)

> **These Conditions Take Time To Turn Around!!** It is very important to understand that even when every step of our treatment that cured my wife was being used- the protocol to down regulate the NO/ONOO cycle, the Earth Calm Home EMF Protection Unit was plugged in (when electrosensitive we have to start at the lowest level so it was a couple of months before we could work up to 'full strength' of protection), almost all in home EMF sources and toxic chemicals were eliminated, pure diet with special nutrients, healing energy work was being done, and so on... for several moths she seemed to be getting weaker and we were not even sure she was making any progress. We simply had no choice but to continue with what we were doing, she then got just well enough to go get Cranial Sacral Therapy that helped complete the process, but thank God we stuck with it all!! **Healing this takes trust in the process and perseverance.**

CHAPTER 3 SUMMARY:

Essentials *__we would do immediately__* if starting over:

1) Start on Dr. Pall's protocol along with additional recommended nutrients: additional selenium, Vitamin B Complex (helpful for ANS too) , Vitamin C, Ecklonia cava (Seanol), Calm (or similar) magnesium/calcium combo
2) Start taking Comprehensive Wellness humic/fulvic product from Mother Earth Labs and Oceans Alive 2.0 Marine Phytoplankton.
3) Obtain Earthing product(s) and 'ground' as many hours per day/night as possible BUT start slow, increasing time.
4) Begin weekly CranioSacral Therapy (CST) treatments, if possible combined with Somato Emotional Release (SER) if able to locate therapists trained in both. *If not able to leave home we would have paid therapist to come to the house and/or use $40 Still Point Inducer from Upledger Institute*
5) Get whole house EMF protection, such as from Earth Calm 'Infinity'. We trust ours to also protect us from smart meters, but for initial healing it is best to have smart meter removed and eliminate use of any wireless, computers, TVs, cell phones, or any other electronic device.
6) Avoid exposure to all toxic chemicals
7) Get a blood nutrition and 'saliva' hormonal test (through Naturopath or DC) and take what is recommended.
8) Balance the Autonomic Nervous System
9) Use mini-trampoline and/or 'chi' type machine for lymph
10) Help Leaky Gut by balancing ANS, Aloe, and G I Sustain

My wife did use all of the above except the humic/fulvic nutritional product (Mother Earth Labs pH Balancer), the Oceans Alive Marine Phytoplankton, and Earthing. By taking humic/fulvic along with the green drinks, whey protein for glutathione production, pure water and a pure diet, and Earthing, it is my belief that the body will usually detox well enough over the course of 4-6 months to be able to heal.

4. OPTIONAL **PRIMARY** TREATMENTS

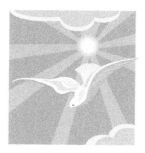

Dynamic Neural Retraining System ?

I feel it important to present this option to consider. We have been hearing a few good, sometimes outstanding results from a few who have tried these methods of 'rewiring' the Limbic system of the brain. The trainings are conducted at live conferences and is available on DVD. These can both be very tricky when someone has severe EMF sensitivity. I suppose for listening to the DVD long wires could be run from the DVD player to speakers.

My understanding of what the developers of the program are saying happens in the case of MCS, CFS, EHS and other similar conditions, is that our autonomic nervous system is in overdrive at all times. [**This is the Sympathetic 'stuck-on' that I have talked about earlier, referred to as the Bowling Ball Syndrome. It may be that correcting this as discussed in Chapter 3 in just a few days will accomplish what they are spending months to do and requires ongoing daily maintenance]**

This programs use a variety of techniques like neuro-linguistic programming, visualizations, meditation, positive affirmations, self-hypnosis, mindfulness, yoga and others to achieve that goal.

Here is an excellent discussion by Cynthia Perkins (looks like she would be a great health coach!) about these programs: http://www.holistichelp.net/limbic-system-retraining.html

Excerpts from the above article:

"Something has gone awry. The limbic system has been damaged or impaired by an "original" toxin or stressor, and now the autonomic nervous system perceives all levels of all chemicals and even items that have no toxicity and all levels of stress as "a threat to survival."

"These programs use a variety of techniques like neuro-linguistic programming, visualizations, meditation, positive affirmations, self-hypnosis, mindfulness, yoga and others to achieve that goal."

"When you are under stress of any kind, be it toxic stress or emotional stress, neurotransmitters in the frontal lobes of the brain like dopamine, serotonin, GABA, endorphins/enkephalins, endocannabinoids histamine are released to modulate the stress response system. Each of these neurotransmitters oppose norepinephrine and therefore turn off the fight or flight system. If there are not adequate neurotransmitters in the brain, then the fight or flight system will not be modulated properly. The sympathetic nervous system will remain dominant.

You should still address any other factors you have going on like nutritional deficiencies, genetic polymorphisms, lyme, bacteria, parasites, or yeast overgrowth etc. that are known to contribute to chemical sensitivities, adrenal fatigue, CFS, etc. You should not be using these brain retraining programs in place of detoxification, proper diet, nutritional supplements etc. Limbic system retraining should be one component of a comprehensive plan, not your sole plan; and let me explain why this is my position."

"Continuing on with our discussion about the autonomic nervous system, here are a few other crucial facts to be aware of.

To successfully rewire the brain or heal an impaired limbic system, you must first have something to work with - neurons and neurotransmitters that work adequately.

Additionally, toxins of all kinds, (pesticides, heavy metals, lyme, bacteria, yeast, sugar, junk food, food additives, air pollution, etc), inhibit the frontal lobes of the brain and prevent adequate neurotransmitter production and function. Since these toxins can cross the blood brain barrier they can land on neurotransmitter and hormone receptors and prevent them from functioning properly. In some cases, they block function, and in other cases, they mimic the natural hormone or neurotransmitter and some do both."

Keep in mind, most people are not even aware that Dr. Tennant let us know about how to get quickly get the body out of 'Sympathetic stuck on', in fact in just minutes, by frequencies to meridian points on the neck with his BioModulator device. I have been able to accomplish the same results using Earthing patches which adds voltage/electrons, just slower, and also with acupuncture patches from Life Wave which are designed to reflect back energy from meridian points and maybe providing the needed frequencies as well. It is certainly worth trying unless you have the $2500 available for the BioModulator. It can be used for all types of healing so it would be a great investment.

So at this time it is unclear to me if there is any advantage to these programs over correcting the Bowling Ball Syndrome, using methods such as Earthing while we sleep and TFT to help keep the Autonomic Nervous System balanced. However we want to see anything that helps people live better lives, and some techniques just resonate better than other for us.

I would still use every other thing I have listed as 'Essential' in Chapter 3 and 7 to help assure a complete and lasting healing.

OPTION S TO USE IN PLACE OF CRANIOSACRAL THERAPY WHEN IT IS NOT AVAILABLE

1) FSM - Frequency Specific Microcurrent
[www.frequencyspecific.com]

Note: For MCS — I would **not** use it while experiencing EMF Sensitivity/EHS at this time. Not enough information yet to feel confident about recommending it for EHS.

"Each cell, tissue and organ has an ideal resonant frequency that coordinates its activities."
-James Oschman, PhD Dover, NH
Author/Co-Author: Body Electric and Energy Medicine- The Scientific Basis

This is a very effective and versatile healing modality that we will be hearing a lot more about in the upcoming years. It is currently used by MDs, Chiropractors, Physical Therapists, Osteopathic Doctors, Naturopaths, and other health professionals. FSM practitioners have a specific protocol they can use for MCS.

What is it? Technically, Frequency Specific Microcurrent therapy is an energy healing therapy using the application of minute amounts of electrical current to specific parts of the body to stimulate self-healing that can dramatically speed the healing process. Microcurrent frequencies have been shown in clinical studies to increase energy (ATP) production in cells by 500%.

FSM was developed by Dr. Carolyn McMakin, using frequencies passed on from an osteopath in Canada who had a practice that came with a machine made in the 1920's. She began developing protocols for the use of frequencies in her clinic to successfully treat chronic myofascial pain resulting in published papers with her clinical results. She began teaching FSM in 1997 to see if the results were reproducible and after seeing that they were her teaching work expanded to what are now three day seminars in the use of different frequency protocols and diagnosis to help patients recover from fibromyalgia, sports injuries, sciatica, and also help with a variety of other conditions such as shingles, brain fog, anal fissures (it healed mine for sure!), and so on.

She is very limited in what she can say FSM will do, however speak with any practitioner using it and I'm sure you will be amazed at the success experienced by their patients/clients.

Dr. McMakin's website is: www.frequencyspecific.com. This is also where you can use a search tool to find a certified practitioner in your area.

I personally experienced incredible results from this therapy when treating both my sciatica and, of all things, an anal fissure which developed during my chemotherapy treatments. We have since learned that in addition to 'microcurrent settings' for MSC, general pain and promotion of healing, there are also settings for a broad range of health conditions such as anxiety, various emotions, heart spasms (used on my wife successfully for heart palpitations!) allergies, and so on. Ask the practitioner to treat the Autonomic Nervous System too! It is a very, very mild treatment, in fact you simply lie on a table and don't really feel anything while it is being administered.

There is an amazing true story conveyed on the FSM website and in Dr. R. Rowan's article (link above) involving the use of FSM on a well-known pro football star. He played for the Philadelphia Eagles the last time that the team was in the Super Bowl.

The remarkable thing that occurred is that this player had a severe ankle injury just weeks before the Super Bowl, which required surgery and the expected recovery time was about 14 weeks. However, he used the Frequency Specific Microcurrent therapy starting immediately after the surgery and throughout his healing, and was able to play in that Super Bowl at almost 100% just 5-6 weeks later! I recall watching that game and his performance with astonishment at how well he was able to play. Only a few years later did I learn about his use of FSM from his story posted on their website after it was recommended to me for helping my sciatica.

How it works

Understanding how specific frequencies can have any effect on the body calls for seeing the body from a quantum perspective of its physical structure rather than by the older mechanical or Newtonian view. When we look down into the tissues of our body, at the subatomic levels, we will find bits of energy vibrating at great speeds. There are electromagnetic bonds holding this energy together. It is also interesting to note that there is far more space being occupied by energy than by matter. This energy can behave in two different ways –like matter or like waves. Understanding the dynamics going on there help explain how past physical and/or emotional trauma can end up energetically remaining in the body long after the body has 'healed' from the initial event.

Dr. James Oschman, PhD is a biophysicist and has published extensively about the scientific basis of energy medicine. [Appendix B, Recommended Reading]

Here are some of his findings:
"In the quantum world classical particles such as electrons are at the same time waves, and waves can do things that particles cannot do" (James Oschman, PhD)

"The cell is filled with a microtrabecular lattice that forms the ground substance within the cell. All of the organelles (very small 'organs' inside of the cellular membrane wall) are suspended and interconnected by the microtrabeculae. Glycoproteins extend across the cell surface from the cell interior to the exterior. These proteins connect with the filamentous network within the cell. The filamentous network is a crystalline gel lined by water molecules and **conveys and stores current, charge and vibrational information**." (James Oschman, PhD 1997)

Then we consider the quote from a Nobel Prize winner: "Molecules do not have to touch each other to interact. Energy can flow through the electromagnetic field….the electromagnetic field, along with water, forms the matrix of life." (Albert Szent-Gyorgyi 1988)

How this all ties in to energetic 'imprinting' and healing: "Every part of the body, including all of the molecules so thoroughly studied by modern science…form a continuously interconnected semiconductor electronic network. **Each component of the organism, even the smallest part, is immersed in a constant stream of vibratory information. Complete health corresponds to total interconnection. Accumulated physical and/or emotional trauma impairs the interconnections. When this happens, the body's defense and repair systems become impaired and disease has a chance to take hold.** Acupuncture and other energy therapies restore balance and vibratory circuitry, with obvious and profound benefits." (James Oschman, PhD)

Based on this evidence, it is not hard to imagine how correcting these stored frequencies in our bodies is often the essential aspect to facilitate true healing. It is now believed that Homeopathy works by providing specific frequencies to help the body heal. Frequency Specific Microcurrent, which can be considered a form of "electronic homeopathy", uses frequencies that closely match the current of the human body and can be fine-tuned to an almost infinite range, depending on what is needed for specific conditions. Clinical trials over years on several thousands of patients have proven that on a clinical level certain frequencies can and do effect specific biological, emotional, and energetic levels in the human body.

I would view Acupuncture, NAET, or NMT as viable options to be part of the core treatment, especially if unable to receive CranioSacral Therapy or Frequency Specific Microcurrent treatments.

2) Acupuncture

Acupuncture is a highly respected and potentially a powerful healing modality. As discussed above in the Frequency Specific Microcurrent discussion, it helps restore and balance the vibratory circuitry to allow the body to function properly. It is particularly effective when performed by a Chinese doctor or someone very skilled and well trained with the ability also read the pulse, eyes and tongue accurately. It is 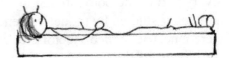 also essential to receive as adequate amount of treatments. Acupuncture was sure a saving grace for my wife at the later stage of my wife's healing. It not only lifted her body's strength and energy but also lifted her spirits enough to get to the next and final stage of her healing journey.

Given enough time, I do think our Chinese Doctor would likely have been able to resolve the sleep, anxiety and heart palpitations, but we seemed to hit a plateau with her response to the treatments. She was starting to get really discouraged since she had already gone through about 5 months of very hard work and lack of good sleep was wearing her down in every way. She also needed to get well enough as soon as possible in order return to work and keep her job of 25 years.

I do think it can only help to add acupuncture along with the other treatments considered as critical or primary, or, it could be used instead of one of them. Either way, starting it right away and with best acupuncturist available would be a great benefit. **Be sure to ask to have the Autonomic Nervous System specifically treated.**

3) NAET - Nambudripad's Allergy Elimination Technique

My wife and I love NAET and our practitioner, Jody. Our experience with NAET convinced me that it has the capability to greatly assist with the effects of MCS and perhaps fully relieve the symptoms. It was NAET treatments that reduced her reactions to environmental chemicals and dusts enough to return to the workplace when her initial chemical sensitivity began after exposure to chemicals and dust in the remodeled building which apparently did not have the fresh air vents opened properly during the winter months. *NAET would probably be the best option for someone who is not 'into' or able to be diligent about following a fairly extensive regimen of supplements while maintaining fairly strict dietary standards for the several months it may take to heal.*

I had been asking around for possible treatments for chemical sensitivities and while at my Network Chiropractor's office getting an adjustment, she connected me with a young lady who was there as a patient to tell me about her experience with NAET. She conveyed that she and her brother had just returned from being in Europe for several months. Both had experienced severe allergies their entire lives to pollens and dusts from nature, and both had reactions so bad they would experience anaphylactic responses. While in Europe, they received NAET treatments and she said they both were completely cured of these allergies.

One of the more fascinating aspects of NAET to me was learning of their belief that many of us are actually 'allergic' to very natural, healthy and necessary things such as vitamins. Added to that, we may have allergic reactions to seemingly inert items like the out-gassing from the plastic of even our 'not brand new' computers and keyboards. While NAET can usually resolve/relieve these 'allergic reactions', and it certainly helped my wife during her first go around with MCS, I believe now that it is the energy/frequency disruptions caused by the 'energy cysts' (discussed in the CranioSacral Therapy and Somato Emotional Release sections) that are the underlying source of the problem and that is the main reason why I give the give the edge to CST and SER over NAET.

The developer of NAET, Dr. Devi Nambudripad, has written a book titled "Freedom From Chemical Sensitivities" which could be very helpful for anyone considering using NAET as either a primary or adjunct treatment.

4) NMT – NeuroModulation Technique

I used this modality while overcoming cancer to assist the body's ability to fight it and to get the most effectiveness from the chemotherapy treatments I was receiving. I believe that combining NMT with Dr. Pall's Protocol may also lead to a complete healing. NMT is a powerful tool to help the mind-body freely realize its potential to heal. It is well worth considering especially if you have a practitioner near you and he/she has a solid reputation.

It is best described as "informational medicine," because it works to identify and correct the informational source of illness - the confusion that can interrupt our innate healing mechanisms. The NMT position is that illness is the inevitable result of informational confusion and faults in the systems responsible for regulating body functions, making them unable to produce the balanced internal-body state that wellness requires.

The mind-body is a self-correcting system that always seeks to find and maintain the balanced internal state in which optimal health and vitality thrive

"The mind-body was created with an amazing intelligence that allows it to produce a fully formed human being from a single cell and to develop into trillions of body cells communicating perfectly to heal the body and maintain vitality throughout its lifespan. When that communication fails, the NMT system is a unique and powerful tool by which the NMT practitioner enters into a carefully developed therapeutic dialog with the patient's mind-

body. NMT uses special routines of questions and corrective training statements that are organized into therapeutic templates known as NMT clinical pathways." www.nmt.md

Bodies suffer all sorts of negative impacts in life: trauma, toxins, infection, stressors including emotional, physical, chemical, malnutrition, and other challenges. Nutritional support, diet, and exercise are all important to help promote healing and prevent healing.

The founder of NMT believes that "no matter what other form of healthcare a patient may choose to receive, if the informational basis of illness has not been addressed, the healing resources of the mind-body simply cannot be applied efficiently."

NeuroModulation Technique website introduction:

http://www.nmt.md/IntroductionToNMT.cfm

You can also locate certified practitioners on their website.

5. MORE GREAT HEALING TOOLS!

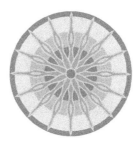

Additional outstanding methods to assist with our well –being, lessen our stress and to promote the healing process.

As mentioned in the introduction, I am telling what we did to 'cure' (heal) my wife and/or what we would now do if we had to start over based on what we learned during my wife's healing journey in an effort to lessen the trauma, decrease the time it might take to heal and lessen the cost. For example, she he did not use TFT which is listed first, but did use something called W.H.E.E (a hybrid of EFT and EMDR) and EFT, which is similar and also very effective. However, TFT would probably now be preferred tapping choice.

1) TFT -Thought Field Therapy   [www.rogercallahan.com]
Please note: While discussed earlier in Chapter 3, this is an in depth look at TFT. Think of TFT as self-administered acupuncture.

This appears to be one of the most effective methods that you can learn to do yourself which is capable of quickly relieving symptoms of stress, anxiety and insomnia which all have an adverse effect on the body's ability to heal. These are common issues facing most people that have MCS and/or EHS. It seems that our body chemistry gets out of sorts with all of the imbalances going on and an escalation of emotions comes along with that.

Excessive stress alone has been attributed to 80% of illnesses we experience in our modern world by leading experts, and this is due primarily to the negative impact on our adrenal glands. Adrenal exhaustion is considered by many health experts to be the primary cause of Multiple Chemical Sensitivities, so reducing stress becomes an area of particular importance for this condition. True healing is also very difficult to accomplish without enough quality sleep.

My wife used EFT, a very similar 'tapping' method, during her healing process and felt it definitely helped her deal better with challenging emotional responses that arose pretty much daily. These emotional states can easily make it much more difficult to maintain the feeling of hope that truly is essential to have in order to keep going through the healing process. I am convinced that having CranioSacral Therapy treatments right at the beginning of healing would drastically lessen the emotional overload by reducing stress, anxiety and insomnia much more effectively by permanently releasing the 'energy cysts' (discussed earlier) which I consider a primary cause of most of the emotional distress.

However, the great thing about WHEE, TFT and EFT is that you can use them on yourself whenever needed. I think any one of these will be very effective and helpful. It is possible that you can find a therapists/counselor that uses one or the other and who's services would be covered by your health insurance, so that may be a deciding factor. I think it is essential to purchase the how-to books for each method and trying them out for and on yourself to see which is most effective for you. I am just learning about TFT and my understanding so far is that EFT is a more simplified version of TFT. While EFT is highly regarded for its effectiveness, TFT is a little more involved to learn, but it may also be more powerful. A nationally recognized figure in the holistic health field, Dr. Joseph Mercola, has very positive opinions of both methods. He has articles published on his web site about each. His current opinion is that EFT is the preferred technique. I think both are excellent and so is the WHEE method. I see that Jack Canfield, author of the Chicken Soup for the Soul book series has given his strong endorsement of TFT.

TFT was developed by Roger Callahan, a student of Emotional Freedom Technique (discussed in next section).

From the TFT website: www.rogercallahan.com

For the past 30 years, a simple technique called Thought Field Therapy has been rapidly healing negative emotions such as trauma and anxiety—and even disease—for people who are desperate to regain wellness and normalcy in their lives.

What started as a simple therapeutic treatment to stimulate the body's own healing systems through the identification of a specific code and then tapping this code on various points of the body—using the same system Chinese acupuncturists do—has become a mainstream therapy accepted by medical doctors, psychologists, alternative healthcare practitioners and even military mental-health personnel.

Thousands of people have recovered rapidly from troublesome disorders like insomnia, gout or tinnitus. Others have eliminated stress, anxiety and phobias such as fear of flying and fear of public speaking—literally within minutes. Still others with life-threatening cancer have completely reversed the disease. Hundreds have regained their lives by curbing addictive urges for nicotine, controlled substances or obsessive behaviors. And those suffering the aftereffects of trauma—warfare, rape, injury or loss—have instantly removed the horrible emotions and feelings tied to that event which previously controlled their lives, sometimes for decades.

A clinical study conducted by Florida State University's Physcosocial Stress Research Program & Clinical Laboratory of four approaches that held promise for treating PSTD. The four approaches were Traumatic Incident Reduction, Visual Kinesthetic Dissociation, Eye Movement Desensitization and Reprocessing (EMDR), and Thought Field Therapy (TFT).

When reporting the results, Charles Figley, PhD stated that the results of all treatments were impressive, however TFT stood out from all other approaches he was aware of because of the following reasons:

1) It is extraordinarily powerful, in that clients receive nearly immediate relief from their suffering and the treatment appears to be permanent.
2) It can be taught to nearly anyone so that clients can not only treat themselves but treat other affected.
3) It appears to do no harm
4) It does not require the client to talk about their troubles, something that often causes more emotional pain and discourages many for seeking treatment.
5) It is extremely efficient (fast and long-lasting).

Additional endorsements for the effectiveness of TFT can be found on:

http://life-excellence.com.au/research.html

http://www.psychotherapy-center.com/tft_what_experts_and_academicians_are_saying.html

2) EFT - Emotional Freedom Technique
[www.eftuniverse.com]

This simple technique, which can be easily self-taught, was probably the most effective self-administered method my wife used to reduce stress, manage emotional distress as it arises, and assist the overall healing process of our Treatment Plan. It has proven its effectiveness in many scientific studies and is endorsed by a number of well-respected and nationally acclaimed professionals such as Deepak Chopra, M.D., author of numerous health and healing books; Dr. Joseph Mercola, recognized for his promotion of natural health and healing; and Bruce Lipton, PhD., author of the widely acclaimed book Biology of Belief.

The method basically involves tapping meridian points on the body while making statements related to the issues you are dealing with. It works on a variety of health issues, psychological problems, and performance issues, even those that have been resistant to other methods. It can be learned and applied rapidly, which has contributed to its popularity among millions of people.

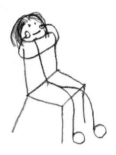

We only learned about it quite late in my wife's healing process and really wish we had known about it all along. She was actually able to find a licensed counselor who teaches and uses EFT during her sessions. I really believe her healing journey would have taken less time and been less intense if she had known about it and used it at the very beginning of her MSC/EHS.

Dr. Joseph Mercola has a good article on his website, www.eft.mercola.com, which, at least as of few months ago, offers a free download of the rather easy to follow, basic how-to EFT instructions. The main EFT website from the founder of the technique is: www.EFTUniverse.com

3) WHEE : Whole Health – Easily and Effectively
[www.wholistichealingresearch.com]

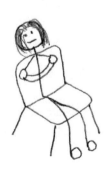

WHEE is a unique and powerful hybrid of EFT and EMDR developed by Dr. Daniel Benor, PhD.

My wife used this technique throughout her healing to very effectively assist with her intense emotional challenges and to address mind/body complications at the times when her (subconscious) mind was the cause of her experiencing symptoms of sensitivities.

Quotes about Dr. Benor's book: **"Seven Minutes to Natural Pain Relief"** *Use for all aspects of healing, not just physical pain*

"Dr. Daniel Benor's book will empower you by giving you the tools with which you can learn from your pain, restore your health and heal your life."
Bernie Siegel, MD author of ***Love, Medicine & Miracles***

"Dr. Benor is both a gifted psychotherapist and a remarkable healer. This book is a must-read as it contains a plethora of insights into the human psyche and very pragmatic approaches to creating patterns of health and well-being in our lives. Dr. Benor's WHEE technique is one of the most effective and efficient methods that I have experienced in alleviating physical and emotional pain and suffering. This is not only a book to read, but something to experience!"
Lucia Thornton, RN, MSN **President, American Holistic Nurses Association**

"Daniel Benor is one of the most creative, inspired healers in our culture. In his latest achievement, he has combined two recognized approaches to pain management and related problems. The result is WHEE, a non-drug, non-surgical technique that is a major breakthrough. This discovery is a gift to the millions of [pain sufferers who are still seeking relief. If pain is a part of your life, you can't afford to not read this book."
Larry Dorsey, MD author of ***The Extraordinary Healing Power of Ordinary Things***

4) EMDR – Eye Movement Desensitization and Reprocessing

This is another quite efficient therapy to release emotional distress from past events to assist in the healing journey. While this therapy requires the assistance of another person, in contrast to WHEE, TFT, or EFT, the utilization of EMDR by Therapists and

Counselors makes this technique more likely to get covered through your health insurance.

We used this therapy for my wife at home during the stage when she was homebound. A dear friend who was experienced with the EMDR process come our house to help. The interesting part of this was that while the standard EMDR technique incorporates a movement of the eyes while following the therapists hand/finger as it moves back and forth during guided talk about a particular event, we learned that using 'tapping', such as tapping on the knees (left, right, left, right...say for 48 times) was just as effective.

She had four sessions this way and they were really powerful. I actually was able to conduct several very powerful sessions with my wife by myself by doing the tapping for her as well as the guided talk therapy. It really is a pretty straight forward process after having experiencing it first hand for several sessions. You first ask the person receiving the EMDR what is the most difficult emotional issue for them at that time, and then, *ask the person exactly where they feel it in their body*. You tell them to stay focused on that feeling in their body and do the tapping a certain number of times, like 48 as described above. You then ask what they feel now and exactly where they feel it in their body. You keep repeating these steps, until there is no longer any emotional distress about the original issue.

From the EMDR International Association website.
www.emdria.org

Eye Movement Desensitization and Reprocessing (EMDR) is an integrative psychotherapy approach that has been extensively researched and proven effective for the treatment of trauma. EMDR is a set of standardized protocols that incorporates elements from many different treatment approaches. To date, EMDR has helped an estimated two million people of all ages relieve many types of psychological stress.

No one knows how any form of psychotherapy works neurobiologically or in the brain. However, we do know that when a person is very upset, their brain cannot process information as it does ordinarily. One moment becomes "frozen in time," and remembering a trauma may feel as bad as going through it the first time because the images, sounds, smells, and feelings haven't changed. Such memories have a lasting negative effect that interferes with the way a person sees the world and the way they relate to other people.

EMDR seems to have a direct effect on the way that the brain processes information. Normal information processing is resumed, so following a successful EMDR session, a person no longer relives the images, sounds, and feelings when the event is brought to mind. You still remember what happened, but it is less upsetting. Many types of therapy have similar goals. However, EMDR appears to be similar to what occurs naturally during dreaming or REM (rapid eye movement) sleep. Therefore, EMDR can be thought of as a physiologically based therapy that helps a person see disturbing material in a new and less distressing way.

Special note regarding 1-4:
*I do believe that CranioSacral Therapy along with the SER mentioned earlier, may be more effective and efficient for releasing emotional distress, however TFT, EFT, EMDR and WHEE discussed above are all outstanding options to use either as an adjunct treatment or, if not able to either find a therapist or afford to have the CranioSacral with SER .

5) Massage

We were extremely grateful for the benefits that massage therapy gave my wife (and me!) during her healing journey. We both really, really looked forward to each session, as they seemed to give us what we needed to keep on going in a better frame of mind. This also was done when my wife was homebound, and it took some effort but we were able to find a wonderful therapist, who came to our home for a very reasonable fee. I find that most people in alternative health field are very kind and generous souls.

Your body is doing a lot of healing and you are likely experiencing a significant amount of anxiety and energetic disarray. Massage can be very helpful in assisting your body to move toxins along and out, helping it with the healing process, and it usually is very mentally and emotionally 'grounding'. Relaxation plays a major role in assisting with the efficiency of the healing process. This has been well established by the medical community. I my view having at least one massage per week during healing would be best, at least during the initial phase where all bodily systems are being severely challenged.

6) Homeopathy

Homeopathy is highly regarded by naturopaths and most holistic practitioners for good reason. It is gentle and yet can be powerful in its positive effects on your physical, mental, and emotional health. When you work with a homeopathic practitioner, the remedies are targeted specifically for you, based on specific information about your health history, your family's health history, your mental and emotional tendencies, and your current symptoms.

I think the key is to be sure to find someone who is very professional, well-trained, and experienced to work with. My wife used someone trained in 'traditional/classical homeopathy'. While the initial consultation may cost somewhere around $150, the overall cost of treatment (the remedies) after that is very low.

7) PSYCH-K [www.psych-k.com]

I was exhilarated by the new realization that I could change the character of my life by changing my beliefs. I was instantly energized because I realized that there was a science-based path that would take me from my job as a perennial "victim" to my new position as "co-creator" of my destiny. (Prologue, xv)"
— *Bruce H. Lipton*

This is a simple, powerful technique to re-program the subconscious mind so it is working for your health and well-being, rather than against it. If you have any doubt about the power of your subconscious beliefs and their effect on your health, please check out the work done by Bruce Lipton, PhD, author of **Biology of Belief: Unleashing the Power of Consciousness, Matter & Miracles**. You can find a series of talks by him on YouTube and I highly recommend getting his book.

His work on this subject is amazing! Several very experienced and knowledgeable holistic health professionals with whom I have shared his book have been 'blown away' by his scientific clarification of this powerful connection between our mind (especially the subconscious mind) and every cell in our bodies. There are a number of other excellent books now available about this subject, but I think everyone should read his work.

Bruce Lipton explains how recent scientific understandings prove that our mind has a direct influence on every cell in the body and that the influence is even more powerful than genetics. He explains why he has come to believe that the subconscious mind is approximately 100 times more influential on our health than our conscious minds.

"There is no need to consider the subconscious a scary, super-powerful, Freudian font of destructive 'knowledge'. In reality, the subconscious is an emotionless database of stored programs whose function is strictly concerned with reading environmental signals and engaging in hard wired behavioral programs, no questions asked, no judgments made. The subconscious mind is a programmable hard drive into which our life experiences are downloaded. The programs are fundamentally hardwired stimulus-response behaviors. The fundamental behaviors, beliefs and attitudes we observe in our parents become 'hardwired' as synaptic pathways in our subconscious minds. Once programmed into the subconscious mind, they control our biology for the rest of our lives...unless we can figure out a way to reprogram them." - Dr. Bruce Lipton, author, The Biology of Belief

The tricky part has been how to reprogram these beliefs. Positive affirmations is one method that has been used, however it relies on the conscious mind and so, even with herculean efforts by the person using positive affirmations, these stand little chance of being successful in overcoming the powerful subconscious programming. Other methods involve the process of encountering unpleasant emotions in an effort to release their mental and physical impact on us.

Psych -K was developed specifically as a way to effectively reprogram those subconscious 'tapes' using a rather simple method. In simple terms, the practitioner uses a specific method to read the body to discover what false or unhealthy beliefs reside in our subconscious and then utilizes specific movements that engage both our left and right brain while stating an affirmation to lock in the new belief. Bruce Lipton has experienced the effects of Psych-K personally and endorses it wholeheartedly as one of the most effective ways to reprogram ourselves for health, and he says happiness too! What a great combination.

Psych-K   [www. psych-k.com]

Book: "Biology of Belief: Unleashing the Power of Consciousness, Matter & Miracles" by Bruce Lipton, PhD

6. THE LIST GOES ON

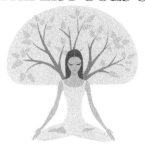

Low cost, effective tools to support healing

There are a number of other excellent healing modalities and treatments available for comfort and relief, or as an adjunct to the primary treatments. We used most of these at some time during my wife's healing process. *Most are available to learn or use at very low cost!*

1) Yoga or Tai Chi

These are two easy to learn, time-tested and easy to use practices that are proven to be very beneficial to overall health and well-being. You can readily find how-to books and or DVDs available at your library or bookstore and learn basic steps yourself. Most communities have very low cost Yoga and Tai Chi classes available in the evenings.

Trust me, when facing the challenges of MCS and/or EHS, tools such as these can be a real asset and may become part of a cherished lifelong routine for you.

2) Music

Here is another simple, inexpensive, science based technique to assist you in dealing with mental and emotional stress, and difficulty falling to sleep, all of which you may be dealing with.

We have just recently hear of music by Mark Romero which is promoted as being able to protect from the effects of EMF in addition to reducing stress and a sense of balance the listener. We look forward to trying his music out real soon by sending it to someone who is challenged by EMFs. [markromeromusic.com]

The CDs we used were made by a researcher, Dr. Jeffrey Thompson who has been producing this type of wave embedded music for over 20 years, working with thousands of patients in clinical research.

Theta waves: During peaceful, meditative states, your brainwave pattern changes to slow-frequency Theta waves. Numerous studies have confirmed that after only a few minutes of listening, your brainwaves naturally lock on to these Theta processes effortlessly transporting you to a deep reflective calm.

Delta waves: In the deepest state of sleep your brainwave patterns change to slow frequency Delta waves, and Dr. Thompson has developed ways to embed these Delta pulses into nature sound recordings. The research has shown that after a few minutes of listening, your brain will lock into the Delta pulses and lead you more easily into deep and restful sleep. www.neuroacoustic.com

More recently a friend with EHS/EMF sensitivity found that a CD called Opening by Heather Noell [heathernoell.com]was very calming, not only for her but she noticed a significant difference with her cats. Just playing it in the background was very effective. Also consider healing music at www.wholetones.com. I just purchased the CDs as MP3 downloads. **We look forward to seeing if others find these helpful.**

3) Qigong

I had heard a number of positive things about Qigong over the years from friends who were either health practitioners or who were just very aware of the healing modalities available. During my wife's healing journey, the close friend who had assisted us so much, loaned us an excellent book written by a Qigong instructor, Master Lin from Minnesota, called "Born A Healer". His story and the message he conveys are quite remarkable, and he has made it a mission to simplify Qigong while preserving its power to heal. He concluded that the typical methods taught through the years have been so overly complicated and not necessary. The book gives a few basic routines which can easily be learned and utilized by anyone, and he calls his method Spring Forest Qigong. He says these are very powerful and they only take a few minutes a day.

While my wife only used a few of the routines a few times, had other healing tools not come along for us, like our Chinese Doctor/Acupuncturists or CranioSacral Therapy, I would have encouraged her to utilize the Qigong more. At one point when we just were not making enough progress on her sleep and heart palpitations, I almost made an appointment at Master Lin's clinic in Minnesota, which would be about a 6 hour drive for us. However, as soon as she started the CranioSacral Therapy, she knew it was making a huge difference and it soon resolved those issues.

I think Dr. Lin is really on to something powerful. I think it is an awesome thing to pursue as a life enhancing strategy as well as something to use as a powerful adjunct in achieving a complete healing of MCS and EHS. *I love simplification and it looks like he has achieved that with the practice of Qigong!* **If learned well and used properly, it may, on its own, be powerful enough to achieve complete healing for many diseases or conditions!**

Master Lin's website: http://www.bornahealer.com

"We in the field of nutrition and medicine have much to learn from healing masters like Chunyi Lin."
   Henry C. Emmons, M.D., Northfield, Minnesota

Master Lin explains that since literally everything is energy, we are energetic beings and every cell in our body is actually a form of energy. He believes thoughts and sickness are also forms of energy.

Energy is known to be constantly transforming and can never be destroyed, but only transformed, and the issue regarding our health is which way our body's energy is transforming –for worse or for better.

He says that in simple terms, Spring Forest Qigong healing is done through manipulating and transforming the energy that is the root cause of an illness. By this transformation of energy it can not only change it to be for the better but can also undo the worst. He says our body is designed to have its energy as always flowing smoothly and in perfect balance. It flows through many energy channels or meridians in the body.

He likens the energy flowing in our body to that of a river. When it is flowing smoothly everything is in balance and is fine. Whenever there is a blockage, problems begin. The water upstream starts overflowing the banks, and downstream the river begins to dry up. Remove the blockage and all returns to normal.

In the same way, Master Lin says, disease is caused by energy blockages in out body resulting in too much or too little energy in one place. He believes these energy blockages are caused by many things but most commonly by emotions or by stress. The blockages then cause the body's natural healing system to malfunction. The energy is not 'good' or 'bad' energy, but rather energy is just energy and the problems only result when there is too much or too little in any given place in our body.

Master Lin says once the blockage or blockages are removed and the energy balance is restored, not the disease, sickness, or other health problems will go away and not only the symptoms, but the root cause of the problem is removed as well.

In summary then, he says that Spring Forest Qigong is a beautiful and powerful way to remove energy blockages to keep the energy flowing smoothly and in balance and this will enable us to live the healthiest, happiest, and most productive and rewarding life possible.

4) Cleansing/detoxing herbs and supplements

Highlights: Humic/Fulvic; adequate voltage and glutathione levels; modified citrus pectin; chlorophyll

The current holistic oriented treatments for MCS focus on cleansing the blood and liver, and attempting to rid the body of stored toxins in fatty tissues. The liver and kidneys need extra support to handle the extra work being done as toxins are released. The theory is that the exposure to these chemicals results in an immune response which results in the body isolating the chemicals (such as storing them in fatty tissue) as a defense mechanism. Over time the body's ability to respond becomes impaired.

We used both herbal and homeopathic remedies to cleanse and support the liver and kidneys along with the de-toxing baths discussed below. It is also very important to use only top quality herbals and homeopathic remedies. What also seems essential is to pace the cleansing to prevent too much stress on the body, which is all too easy to do. I think it is best to error on the side of going slower than necessary. We prefer to either go very slow, or to work closely with trained professional, such as with a Naturopath, on your cleansing work. This would also be a great source for getting professional grade supplements.

While we did not learn of this early enough to use it, one of the more intriguing supplements for mild, safe de-toxing of heavy metals is *modified* citrus pectin (it must be modified so it will bind to the toxins), which acts as a chelating agent. Clinical evidence has shown it to be extremely effective. Many health experts believe that the accumulation of these heavy metals to which we all have had heavy exposure, is a primary factor causing health problems and eliminating them safely is necessary for healing. As mentioned earlier, there is always a real concern about de-toxing too rapidly and over taxing the kidneys or liver which can actually lead to a worsening of health.

We have also since learned about the remarkable detoxing qualities of the Humic/Fulvic that is the base item in the pH-Balancer product we would use from Mother Earth Labs as one essential components for healing MCS and EMF Sensitivity. It provides the charge needed on cell walls to allow nutrients to get in the cell and the toxins to get flushed out. There is plenty of research available that verifies this. See motherearthlabs.com.

Concerned about mercury toxicity? In Hungary a study was done with Humic/Fulvic to see how well it could remove mercury from the organs of pigs. From an article by Dr. Robert Rowan, MD in the Second Opinion Newsletter on July 1, 2006: (the substance from Peat discussed below is Humic)

"Last month, I told you about an inexpensive Hungarian supplement made from peat. I also told you about the miraculous way this supplement draws heavy metals out of your body.

What is most amazing about this supplement, though, is that it can pull certain heavy metals out of your body that we thought were impossible to remove.

Take mercury, for instance. Mercury is the toughest common toxic metal to grab and remove. Even IV chelation therapy doesn't do much to pull mercury out of your body. But look at what happens when you use peat.

In a recent study, researchers looked at how well they could remove mercury from pigs, an animal with very similar detoxification to humans. They divided 15 pigs into three groups of four and a fourth group of three. The researchers acclimated the pigs for five days on a standard diet. Then they gave each pig a *measured dose of radioactive mercury in its feed. And, finally, they administered a **humic/fulvic** acid complex to groups two through four in increasing doses. So group four received a higher dose than groups two and three.*

The researchers measured radioactive mercury in their feces and urine each day. The animals in group four, which received a full dose of the complex, excreted 86% of the ingested mercury compared to 64.9% in controls.

During the 11 days of the trial, the complex caused a 21% increase in mercury elimination.

But the good news doesn't stop there. The researchers then measured residual mercury in the pigs' organs. In the full-dose animals, there was a fall in mercury in all organs examined (including kidney, liver, lung, testicles, skeletal muscle, and brain). The reduction was statistically significant in brain, kidney, and lung. The brain had a whopping 87% reduction in mercury, as compared to controls!"
    Dr. Robert Rowan, Second Opinion Newsletter July, 2006

It is interesting to note that Dr. Jerry Tennant, author of "Healing is Voltage" stresses that the body having adequate voltage (electrons) is very important before starting a detox. I believe that using 'Earthing' devices while sleeping is an excellent way to help assure that. He states that low voltage is usually a sign of a poorly functioning thyroid. Dr. Tenant also emphasizes that the body having an adequate supply of glutathione especially while detoxing is equally important because it is the 'director of detoxification.

Extra quantities of the green drinks already suggested in Part 1 are especially beneficial during any cleansing. The chlorophyll they contain in significant quantities has numerous health benefits and has been identified by the medical community as being capable of removing heavy metal buildup because it can bind with heavy metals to remove them. A recent U.S. Army study revealed that a chlorophyll-rich diet doubles the life-span of animals exposed to radiation.

We often refer to "Healthy Healing" by Linda Page, N.D. for additional guidance on de-toxing as well as guidance for any health concerns.

5) De-toxing baths

Two great ways to assist the cleansing work are detoxing baths and saunas. There are a number of ways to make a bath detoxing and far more beneficial to your health and most are very inexpensive. Remember, if you have city water, please be aware that your water is almost sure to contain chlorine and you will absorb it into your body from showers or bathing. The chlorine is toxic to you. I highly recommend getting de-chlorinating filter for your bath water, like one called Splish Splash by Enviro Products. It will de-chlorinate about 200 baths and costs around $40. Why be adding any toxins to your body when you are working so hard to get them out.

One example of an inexpensive yet effective bath is dissolving 8 oz. of typical baking soda in your bath water and simply soaking for 30 minutes.

Clay baths are another powerful way to detoxing the body. We used products from L.L. Magnetic Clay and I highly recommend going to www.magneticclay.com and learning about the different clays available for everything from Radiation to Formaldehyde and Mercury. My wife took a number of baths for Radiation and Formaldehyde to assist her specifically with the MCS and EHS.

Please note that L. L. Magnetic Clay suggests that you do not use a full bath, if your body is too 'acidic', meaning that your PH is not alkaline enough. They suggest starting with foot baths instead. You can test your PH by wetting special strips with your saliva that will change its color and then matching the color chart to determine the PH. Apparently they believe the bath could be too powerful if our PH is not in a healthy enough range. We took the advice

I give the company a lot of credit for this ethical guidance since it results in using less clay for the foot baths and requires much more patience by their customer.

You (or a friend/family member) can go online or go to your local health food store to get information about how to best correct your PH balance. There are lists available of foods and drinks that are acidic and reduce your PH or are alkaline and will increase your PH. I know it is not easy to accomplish for most of us. My wife was so determined to get well and, to her credit , she was very disciplined and she was very successful in quickly getting her PH in the range suggested by the company to use the clay baths.

Food grade Hydrogen Peroxide – 35% food grade H 2 O2, can also be used for detoxing baths. Nationally acclaimed author Linda Page, N.D. recommends 1 cup in the bath and soaking for 30 minutes.

Linda Page also highly recommends using dried seaweeds from your health food store (or buy on the internet) in the bath water to detox, stimulate lymph drainage, and boost the adrenals (especially good because you are likely dealing with adrenal fatigue).

My wife also took a number of cleansing baths using a special mineral 'oxygenated' soap and a mineral 'neutralizer' which is typically used for consumption, from the company NatureRich [www.naturerich-inc.com]. These were highly recommended by our dear friend who has assisted so many others in their natural healing process. The baths were quite an experience for my wife. They were very soothing yet very powerful. She would feel very warm for a long time after each one. I believe that was due to the internal 'oxygenating' that was happening and my understanding is that getting oxygen to our cells is very desirable for healing.

Again, my thought based on our experience, is to proceed cautiously and be very careful not to do too much too fast, which will tax the body and possibly create more problems. You can decide to be directed by your own response, or consider using 'muscle testing' techniques to read your energetic response (inner intelligence) to help determine 'if, what types of bath, and how often', or consult your Naturopath for guidance. In general, I would say start out slow, one detox bath per week, and stay less time in the bath at first. I guess the expression 'baby stepping' is another way to put it.

6) Saunas

Both conventional saunas and the newer Far Infrared saunas are known to be very effective for releasing toxins from the body and offer a number of other potential health benefits. I am particularly intrigued by recent research on the Far Infrared type. The fact that a highly respected integrative cancer treatment center, the Block Integrative Cancer Center in Illinois, plans to have these available as part of their care for cancer patients, makes a powerful statement about their value. The founder and director, Dr. Keith Block, is also Director of Integrative Medicine at the University of Illinois and is very thorough in all of his research. His book on cancer care, "Life Over Cancer" is an invaluable resource for powerful self-care information for any one with cancer. I found it to be extremely helpful to me when overcoming the cancer in my own body a couple of years ago.

My concern about using saunas is that it is very easy to do too much de-toxing too fast. It is very, very easy to stress the body too much when the body is already being challenged with MCS and/or EHS. I think proceeding cautiously is the best way to go, and if in doubt, just don't use them at all during your crisis time. Staring with 10 minutes sessions at a lower heat , several days apart, and gradually working up. have no doubt that they can be an outstanding addition to our health healing and maintenance.

7) Moderate exercise

It is universally accepted that movement is healthy for the body. It is so valuable for getting oxygen and nutrients to our cells, and getting wastes and toxins moved along to get flushed out. My wife's guidance from our healing friend was to exercise moderately - primarily by walking (outside if possible) and dancing. However she was to avoid anything strenuous. Even use of our rebounder (mini trampoline) would have been too intense for her. Yoga and Tai Chi would also be an excellent, inexpensive ways to accomplish the goals of movement with moderation.

8) Spiritual nurturing

I think we always need to incorporate the 'Spirit' in the healing mix. Mind, Body, and Spirit are what we all know to be the regarded as the essential elements of holistic health and healing. They are much like legs of a stool. All three are necessary for support. We know that if one leg is too short (neglected) the stool is unstable.

Here are some ways we have to nurture our spiritual self: music, meditation, connection with nature, art, Holy Scripture, prayer, inspirational movies and books, Yoga, Tai Chi, funny movies, all laughter, and special time with friends and family.

9) Chakra opening and balancing

Chakras are understood to be energy centers in our body. Our bodies are made of molecules composed of atoms which are made of energy. Those who work with these energy centers have learned that having the chakras open and balanced are an essential component of maintaining mental, emotional, spiritual and physical health. Measurements have confirmed there are concentrations of energy (voltage) right in these areas.

For the past twenty years, Valerie Hunt, a professor of kinesiology [the study of human movement], has measured human electromagnetic output under different conditions. Using an electro-myograth, which records the electrical activity of the muscles. Hunt, like Dr. Hiroshi Motoyama [scientist and Shinto priest], recorded radiations emanating from the body at the sites traditionally associated with the chakras. Through her research she made the startling discovery that certain types of consciousness were related to certain frequencies.

We use a simple and effective method to open and balance our chakras. With each step below, count to 9 or say a 'mantra' or other favorite spiritual phrase 9 times in your head or out loud.

- Hold your left ankle lightly with one hand and left knee with the other hand, repeat the phrase (mantra) with the intention that the energy between your knee and ankle flow easily.
- Now lightly grasp your left knee and left hip and repeat same.
- Hold right ankle and right knee and repeat mantra (or count).
- Now grasp right knee and right hip and repeat mantra (or count).
- Next, place hands on each hip and repeat mantra (or count).
- Now place one hand on the first (Root) chakra (lap or groin area) and other hand just above it on the 2nd (Sacral) chakra, repeat mantra (or count).
- Move lower hand to the third (Solar Plexus) chakra just over the other hand and just above the navel, leaving the other hand in place on the 2nd chakra and use count or say mantra.
- Next take lower hand and place it over the 4th (Heart) chakra, at heart level and count or say mantra
- Now place lower hand on your throat for the 5th (Throat) chakra and repeat mantra (or count).
- Place lower hand on your forehead where the 6th (Third Eye) Chakra is located, again leaving other hand in place on the throat area and repeat your counting or mantra.

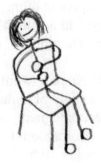

- Leaving one hand on your forehead, place the other on the top of your head on the 7th (Crown) chakra and repeat count/mantra.
- Leaving on hand on top of your head, take the other and hold it above your head, with palm turned upward and do count/mantra.
- Lastly, take the other had from your head and hold it above head with palm faced up so you know have both hands face up above your head and repeat your counting or mantra.

7. PUTTING IT ALL TOGETHER

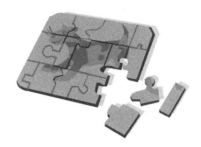

My wife's healing was done by what might be referred to as a shotgun approach, throwing everything at it that seemed viable. We were under a great deal of pressure to find solutions early on just so we could stay in our house, or any typical house. We also needed to maintain enough stability to continue with treatments we had started and incorporate others as were finding them (though my feverish investigation). My wife's fear level was also quite high, most likely exacerbated from the chemical condition occurring with her body's NO/ONOO cycle being spiked - the biological condition which happens to also appear be responsible for Post-Traumatic Stress Disorder according to Martin Pall's work.

I don't regret anything we used and I believe just about everything was helpful. We are deeply grateful for the benefits she did receive from them as they were truly what got her through the tough spots- along with intense prayer and the spiritual support of friends and family. It is only after getting through it that we could see what approach would have been most effective. I am convinced that some treatments, such as CranioSacral Therapy, used right from the beginning would have drastically reduced the need for most of the treatment methods that were used. We see now that most of them were primarily for managing the secondary effects of her illness, like the anxiety, emotional distress, persistent insomnia and heart palpitations. I believe now that they were releasing 'energy cysts' from her body 'little by little' over time. This was an emotionally and physically difficult way to go for her.

It does seem apparent to me that any true healing requires a multi-prong approach that not only addresses all major areas of our health – Physical, Mental (mind/body), Emotional (mind/body), and Spiritual– but will also allow for the reality that we are inherently unique in each of these areas.

The final results of our intense research along with my wife's remarkable courage and diligence to fully implement whatever was deemed as viable, and along with the extraordinary help of our 'extra' ordinary dear friend, was a complete healing, or 'cure' of her severe MCS and EHS.

The way I look at healing these afflictions is really not much different than it would be for healing any illness or condition. It is holistic in the truest sense. Not diagnosing an exact cause. Not attacking anything – with the caveat of putting out the fire of the NO/ONOO cycle, just as we would need to do first in the case of pneumonia, etc. There are numerous theories about what the 'cause' of MCS or EMF sensitivity is, and approaches that try to address these particular aspects. For a few, that may work, but it is quite apparent that the success rate for curing these afflictions has been abysmal at best. I don't think it works when the approach becomes a 'guessing game' by focusing on only one or just a few suspected 'causes'.

Based on what I know now, here is a recap of what I think would be the effective ways to heal/cure MCS and/or EHS:

Essentials:

1) **Martin Pall's (PhD) supplement protocol for several months, plus Seanol, Vit. C, Vit. D3 and B Complex (heavy on B12) (options to Dr. Pall's protocol: Oceans Alive**

Marine Phytoplankton along with Fisetin; possibly 'Epic' by Systemic Formulas) *pages 28-33*

WHY: down regulate the NO/ONOO cycle, support ANS

2) **Earthing (powerful health benefits from efficient grounding of our body to the Earth; added voltage for healing)** *pages 41-44*

WHY: For needed electrons/voltage, Antioxidant, protection from EMF, supports good HRV/Autonomic Nervous System balance, clears blood Rouleaux (undesirable clumping of cells)

3) **CranioSacral Therapy (combined with Somato Emotional Release when possible)** *pages 33-40*

WHY: Restore healthy flow of cerebrospinal fluids to brain and nervous system (this fluid is critical to deliver nutrients and flushes away toxins), helps balance Autonomic Nervous System, removes energetic disturbances (energy cysts)

4) **Correct Sympathetic stuck-on ('Bowling Ball Syndrome') with Tennant Biomodulator, or Earthing patches, or Life Wave Energy Enhancer patches.** *pages 68-72*

WHY: Fastest way to get the body out of 'sympathetic dominance' (fight or flight mode) so Parasympathetic Nervous System can function as it should and help heal the body

5) **Avoidance and/or Mitigation of toxic chemicals and EMF.** *pages 44-54*

WHY: Every exposure impedes healing and can worsen the already out of control NO/ONOO Cycle, toxins stress the body.

6) **pH Balancer from Mother Earth Labs.** *pages 62-64*

WHY: For comprehensive fully bio-available nutrition and detox of chemicals and heavy metals from deep in the tissue; alkalizing

7) Healthy alkalizing diet and pure water (diet includes high quality green drinks and non-denatured whey protein) *pages 59-67*

WHY: An alkalized body promotes health, green drinks for broad based nutrition and helping detox, whey protein to help assure the body has what it needs produce adequate glutathione (the 'master antioxidant' and 'director of detoxification')

8) TFT-Thought Field Therapy or EFT, WHEE, or EMDR *pages 71-72*

WHY: For clearing energy blockages from emotional or physical traumas, TFT for dramatic positive improvement of HRV (Autonomic Nervous System balance), reduces stress that impedes healing

7) Use 'chi' machine or 'rebounder'(mini trampoline) *page 73*

WHY: To get lymphatic system flowing, chi machine helps balance Autonomic Nervous System functioning.

8) De-toxing/calming baths (clay baths, baking soda baths) *Pages 108-110*

WHY: High quality clay baths are very effective at removing toxins, baking soda promotes pH and has a calming effect and provides mild detoxing

9) Testing/treating body chemistry functioning and/or hormonal imbalances (use saliva hormonal and blood nutrition test) *pages 54-57*

WHY: Correcting any significant hormonal imbalance right away will have a dramatic impact on promoting healing, shorten healing time and save money

Remember: *__These are very challenging conditions to turn around and heal from even when you have implemented all aspects listed. In many case it may be a few months to even begin noticing any improvement as the body is doing all it can to put the brakes on the decline, and begin turning the tide at which time healing can be noticed. This take real grit and persistence, however I am confident that by doing all things listed our body will move toward a deep and lasting healing as it did for my wife!__*

Essentials on a tight budget:

Allergy Research Group Nutritional Support Protocol [based on Martin Pall's work] to down regulate the NO/ONOO cycle
OR:
Oceans Alive 2.0 Marine Phytoplankton, also take Fisetin and pH Balancer from Mother Earth Labs (lower cost, possibly easier to tolerate)

Earthing (powerful health benefits from efficiently grounding of our body to the Earth- (as low as $40 for Earthing body bands)

Correct Sympathetic stuck-on ('Bowling Ball Syndrome') with Earthing patches ($20) or Life Wave Energy Enhancer patches ($70)

Avoidance and/or mitigation of chemicals and EMF (Earthing protects from EMF)

Healthy Alkalizing diet and pure water (including whey protein and quality green drinks)

Mini-trampoline $40) or 'chi' type machine ($100

Bach's Rescue Remedy - for calming, emotional support   ($15)

De-toxing/calming baths - baking soda; clay baths   ($3-35)

Use both of these in <u>addition to and/or in place of</u> CranioSacral and Somato Emotional Release when not an option:

TFT -Thought Field Therapy or WHEE (book for one of these- approx. $15)

Still Point Inducer ($30 apparatus to provide fundamental CranioSacral Therapy benefits daily at home)

Add one or more:

Tai Chi, Yoga, and or Qigong (Spring Forest Qigong book-$15-20)

Chakra opening/balancing (free)

Music – Delta and Theta brainwave CDs (CD $15)

- Health insurance may cover CranioSacral Therapy when performed by a Chiropractor or by a Physician. Chiropractic care is always beneficial with healing so it would be a great addition. Massage may be covered if prescribed by a physician and would also be a great addition to the healing process.

Alternatives to use in place of CranioSacral/SER if not an option (from the Essentials list):

Upledger Still Point Inducer – use every day ($40)

For MCS Only: Frequency Specific Micro-current - (if available and able to go out of the house and to practitioner)

TFT-Thought Field Therapy (powerful beneficial effects on balancing the Autonomic Nervous System and stress reduction)

NAET (Nambudripad's Allergy Elimination Technique) for MCS

Acupuncture (highly skilled practitioner)

NMT (NeuroModulation Technique)

Free or almost free, self-taught, very effective healing tools

TFT – Thought Field Therapy

EFT – Emotional Freedom Technique

W.H.E.E. (Hybrid of EMDR and EFT developed by Dr. Daniel Benor, M.D)

Chakra Opening/Balancing

Yoga or Tai Chi

Qigong

Music Therapy

Meditation

Art Therapy

Natural 'Earthing' – bare feet directly contacting the Earth (grass, soil, etc.)

Earthing – products for about $50 will do the job!

HeartMath (* requires initial moderate expense)

8. GOING FORWARD

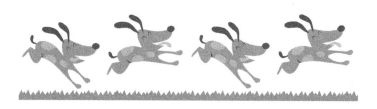

Transitioning back to normal life and staying well

For my wife, knowing she was well enough to resume activities and making the transition back to fully engaging in all aspects of life and work was really the final phase of her healing. It required courage, patience and utilization of a few key tools that have been discussed earlier, such as WHEE and EFT and TFT 'meridian tapping'. Having the support of a professional therapist (who actually taught her the EFT tapping) was very helpful during this time too. Going forward, being grateful always for her recovery and staying well are her primary goals.

The realization that the mind-body connection could have kept her in a never ending loop of the belief she still had chemical and EMF sensitivity even after the physical healing was done, was such a critical aspect of her resuming that normal life. This is discussed more in the pages ahead.

I am very confident that she can stay free of any problems with MCS of EHS for the remainder of her life by the ongoing use of the same powerful healing tools that cured her. This will be much easier to do now that we have discovered so much about this illness and health in general. Maintaining health certainly requires less effort than healing from a crisis state. Now that she is strong with healthy Adrenal Glands (we confirmed her adrenal health with saliva hormonal testing) and appears to have removed most or all of her underlying lifelong stressors (e.g. clearing energy cysts; chemically detoxified), her 'ounce of prevention' will likely be equal to a 'pound of cure'.

Testing the waters

As my wife began to feel more herself in March of 2011, she started inching her way back to normalcy by engaging in activities such as resuming watching a little TV (still shielded to reduce EMFs), visiting and playing card games at the kitchen table with our awesome Granddaughter, and by the end of April she began going to the store for a quick purchase. She was testing the waters, since these activities had been out of the question for over three months during the height of her sensitivity.

Remember that the EMFs from the TV /satellite receiver had previously caused reactions such as tingling in her legs and a general wooziness even with the shielding. Also, being in close proximity of others who had used standard laundry detergent and/or fabric softeners would cause a reaction in her lungs. Going out to 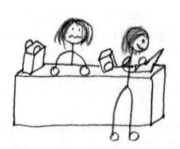 any place of business also means exposure to cell phones, wireless emissions, fluorescent lighting and so on, which had all caused a reaction of flu-like weakness both at our home and also during her last real outing in December 2010.

Mind/Body connection:

It was during this transition time that my wife had several occasions of experiencing the mind/body connection first hand.

Her memories of her reactions and fears associated with reacting to chemicals and EMFs along with the awareness that these reactions would cause a setback in her recovery made her prone to having what felt to her to be physical reactions in certain circumstances when it soon was discovered that her mind was now creating the response and was triggered by her past anxieties. *What she was feeling were real physical symptoms, however, now the cause was different – it was no longer a physical reaction by her body to the environment.* When her 'health coach' (our dear friend) helped her realize this connection was the likely culprit, she was told to use the WHEE and or EFT tapping methods whenever she thought a reaction was starting to occur.

The first encounter:

Her first test with this was when she allowed close contact with family members whose clothes had been laundered by standard detergent with plenty of fragrance and perhaps fabric softener sheet odors and chemicals as well. Keep in mind that her sense of smell, which according to Martin Pall's research (www.thetenthparidigm.org) can become over 100 times more sensitive than normal when the OH/ONOO cycle is really out of control, was still a little more heightened than normal so it was a strong smell to her where it might not be to others.

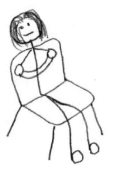

So when she started feeling like she was reacting to the chemicals, she excused herself from the room for a few minutes, did the WHEE tapping and returned. Now, there was no reaction to the chemicals! Just like that....gone. This would not have been possible had the reaction been a physical one as it had been previously. It was clearly being triggered by the memory and anxieties about reacting before and the consequences of those reactions. While in no way suggesting that what soldiers in battle need to endure is comparable to what my wife went through, I do see a similarity with the soldiers who, long after leaving the battlefield and living in a safe environment, will experience intense physical and mental reactions to the sounds of gunshots or explosions, as if they were still in imminent danger.

Experiencing this mind/body connection so clearly and confirming that MCS and EHS reactions/responses, when based only from the mind-even when they seem to be physical - can be stopped almost immediately, was both enlightening and empowering and proved to be pivotal in resuming a normal life for my wife.

Another milestone:

Her next significant experience with using the WHEE and/or EFT to short circuit a mind generated response was when she volunteered to help one hour per week at the local small town library . This turned out to be an excellent way to take the next step back into normal life activities since she would just be there an hour or so once a week and in doing so be exposed to computers, wireless, cell phone, perfumes, paper dusts, cleaning chemicals, etc.

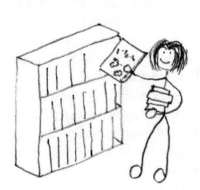

Not surprisingly, her first day triggered some 'reactions', that is until she did the WHEE tapping for a few minutes and found she was able to successfully stay the whole time and really enjoy it. It sure felt great to her to be back in a normal environment with people and office type equipment. She also happens to love being in libraries. After a few times she found that she would stay close to two hours instead of the one she committed to and was not even anxious to leave. *What a great joy for her!! She knew she was going to be able to return to life!! At this stage, her success was all due to her knowing how to overcome the undesirable aspect of the mind/body connection through tapping methods.*

The final and best milestone!

During the depths of her illness, my wife understandably could not imagine being able to return to work even though it was her heart's desire. Besides wanting to work and being incredibly conscientious about her work obligations, being able to do so would also represent the final stage in her healing and a real victory over the Multiple Chemical Sensitivity and EMF Sensitivity (EHS: Electro-Hypersensitivity).

In August 2011, after finally getting the heart palpitations to stop and seeing a dramatic improvement with sleeping (primarily from the CranioSacral and Frequency Specific Microcurrent treatments which she was now able to travel out of the home and receive), she felt it was time to attempt the return to her job and workplace. Her experience volunteering at the library helped give her confidence.

Ironically, a major remodeling of her entire office area had just been completed about 6 months prior, meaning new carpet (probably glued to the floor), new paint, etc. To make this transition, her health coach friend recommended that she go into the office during off hours, evenings and weekends, before her start date and spend an hour or so there and to use the WHEE or EFT tapping at the first sign of what seemed to be a reaction to the chemicals and/or EMFs. Sure enough, the first couples of times she did have the experience of what seemed to be a physical reaction, then she did the tapping and it stopped. The last time she went in she had no reaction and so she felt ready to start out a few hours a day to gain her confidence that she actually would be okay and that she was healed enough to gradually resume full-time 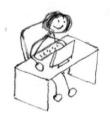 hours. Well, it is currently (as I write this) October of 2012 and she has been working full- time successfully, with no reactions, since September of 2011! She is so very grateful every day to be physically able to work in a normal setting again!

There have been a few rare occasions to this day when she suspects she may be feeling some response to EMF or chemicals, but every indication is that these are from the remnants of the mind/body issue and there is no evidence that the response is physically generated. These things are difficult to say with 100% certainty, however the fact that any time she uses the 'tapping' methods they go away, along with the fact that they are occurring so rarely and far less frequently over time, are strong indications that all is well.

Besides being able to successfully be at the workplace, in the past year she and I have also flown to Washington D.C. and Florida, stayed in hotels and rode in rental cars – all with no problem, no reaction to EMF or chemicals! This is an amazing turnaround, almost unimaginable to the tens of thousands who suffer with these afflictions for years, often while getting worse as time goes on.

Staying Well:

Going forward, I am extremely confident that with reasonable diligence, my wife will not ever need to experience any symptoms of Multiple Chemical Sensitivity or Electro-Hypersensitivity. Little by little, my wife is beginning to believe this as well.

We have new knowledge about the powerful healing modalities available that can keep stress and its effects on the body at a minimum and about the essentials of diet and nutrition.

Based on all that we have learned, here is an overview of how we plan to maintain her excellent health and keep her free of the awful illness that turned our lives upside down and filled her with the fear of never having anything close to a normal life again:

Our MCS and EHS Prevention Plan:

- Maintain a healthy diet which is primarily alkalizing and has sufficient saturated fats. The focus is on fresh fruits, properly prepared fresh or frozen vegetables (organic if possible); small amounts of whole grains; nuts and seeds; organic eggs, butter and plain yogurt ; ground flaxseed and flaxseed oil, coconut oil, olive oil and chia seeds; minimal intake of sugars which are not from eating whole fruits. Stevia will be used as a sweetener. Using our NutriBullet juicer/processor is a super easy way to enjoy fruits and vegetables and in theory making the nutrients more bioavailable.

- Drink purified water using in-home reverse osmosis unit most often with Crystal Energy drops added.

- Take essential supplements regularly: Mother Earth Labs Humic/Fulvic pH Balancer, Vitamin B complex; Essential Fatty Acids; Seanol (brown seaweed extract); quality Green Drinks that contain a variety of organic green foods and multiple antioxidants (extracts of mushrooms, berries, etc.); whey protein powder, Vitamin D3, and Mother Earth Labs Lugol's Iodine Plus (iodine and potassium iodide plus needed cofactors), quality marine phytoplankton Oceans Alive 2.0.

- Continue to minimize exposure to chemicals and EMFs in the home. This is good general practice for everyone and has health benefits beyond prevention of chemical or EMF sensitivities. Use no toxic cleaners or air fresheners in the home; no toxic sprays outside; keep using Earth Calm Whole House Protection unit to mitigate EMF effects, using a hands free headset for cell phones; use of shielding over the computer monitor; no wireless in the house; no electronic devices near the bed; no cordless phone use; etc.

- Earthing all night using Earthing pillowcases or sheet.

- Continue going for regular CranioSacral Therapy treatments. Six per year might be adequate, but we hope she gets them more frequently for now.

- Receive at least 4 or 5 Chiropractic treatments per year, preferably from a 'Network' Chiropractor (Network is a particular technique/method)

- Use EFT, WHEE, or TFT for the initial handling any emotional challenges that arise during the course of life. The CranioSacral treatments will most likely address the stress more thoroughly and prevent it from ever building up to any level of concern.

- Ongoing spiritual self-nurturing both at home and with a broader community

* Special note: We think acupuncture is another excellent option to assist with maintaining health and would always be considered by us as a very viable option

9 FINAL THOUGHTS

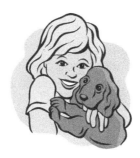

By all accounts, my wife's healing in such a relatively short time period sure has the feeling of a miracle when compared to the experiences of most everyone else facing the type of health challenges that she did. I think the real miracle was that we found the right treatments and combination of them to resolve (or cure) her illness.

In what seems to be a typical pattern in life, the miracle came as a result of an all-out effort to leave no stone unturned in my search for a cure, and my wife's remarkable and heroic dedication to using whatever was deemed worthy to try. The round-the-clock, selfless support and guidance from our dear friend made surviving this possible for us. The use of various healing modalities and the Earth Calm Home EMF Protection Unit gave the time for Dr. Pall's protocol to work, and the combination of all we did helped her become well enough to go and get the CranioSacral Therapy and Frequency Specific Microcurrent treatments that turned out to be what facilitated the last phase of her complete healing.

It amazes me that we used so many healing methods. We are forever grateful for the benefits received by each one and we attribute them to enabling her to make it through the crisis. A special acknowledgement goes to the powerful group healing sessions which moved my wife forward a great deal in developing her belief that she really could get well .We are also very grateful for the remote energy sessions that helped her get through many especially tough stretches when her body, mind and emotions were not serving her well. While I am convinced there is a scientific explanation for how these sessions work, we probably do not yet have enough understanding of the energetic world. In quantum physics there is the term 'entanglement' 'used to describe the energetic connections over a great distance that have been proven to exist. We also think of these methods as being like another form of prayer. We do know that they were a true Godsend to my wife at the time.

In the end, it is my belief that the wisest choice for us when it comes to our healing is that we always should use the very best, most effective methods available. This book attempts to summarize what I believe to be the most effective methods and what approach we would take if starting over with her healing.

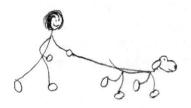

Along with using the best methods available to us, the other essentials to heal seem to be (1) Having the conscious and unconscious belief that we are worthy of being healed (2) That we truly have a desire to live, and (3) We never lose hope. To address these aspects, I would use spiritual practices and PHYCH-K as primary tools. Also, the use of the CranioSacral Therapy, especially when combined with SER (SomatoEmotional Release), is very effective at releasing undesirable energy patterns (energy cysts) which I believe play a significant role in our subconscious belief patterns.

Our deepest wish now is that the trials my wife had to endure has resulted in knowledge that will dramatically lessen, and even end the suffering for others who are facing the severe, debilitating and alarming consequences of Multiple Chemical Sensitivity and/or Electro-hypersensitivity(sensitive to EMFs).

May God bless you in your healing journey.

The Author invites you to share your experience of living with and healing Multiple Chemical Sensitivity and/or EMF Sensitivity [Electro-Hypersensitivity].

Gary's Health Corner
P.O. Box 277
Deerfield, WI. 53531-0277

Facebook page: www.facebook.com/MCSandEMFsensitivitycured

Appendix A

Recommended websites:

Dr. Martin Pall, PhD EMF- NO/ONOO Research article:
http://aaemconference.com/pall.html

Earthing
www.earthinginstitute.net

CranioSacral Therapy / Somatic Emotional Release
www.upledger.com
www.craniosacraltherapy.org
www.mindandbeyond.net

Frequency Specific Microcurrent
www.frequencyspecific.com

General Health
www.tennantinstitute.net
www.drbrownstein.com
www.secondopinionnewsletter.com

PHYCH-K
www.psych-k.com

WHEE
www.wholistichealingresearch.com/whee_process_1

EMF/EHS information
www.bioinitiative.org/freeaccess/report/index.htm
www.electrohypersenitivity.org
www.earthcalm.com
www.weepinitiative.org
www.ei-resource.org
www.hesse-project.org

www.emfwise.com/precautions.php
www.electrosensitivesociety.org
www.emffacts.com

MCS
http://www.mcs-america.org/
http://www.ei-resource.org/
http://www.chemicalsensitivityfoundation.org/
http://bcn.boulder.co.us/health/rmeha/index.htm
http://www.holistichelp.net/multiple-chemical-sensitivity.html
http://www.ciin.org/

NAET-Nambudripad Allergy Elimination Technique
www.naet.com

Network Chiropractic
www.associationfornetworkcare.com

NMT-NeuroModulation Technique
www.nmt.md/IntroductionToNMT.cfm

Chakra information
www.chakrasbalancing.com
www.universal-mind.org/Chakra_pages/ProofOfExistence.htm
www.binaural-mind.com/binaural-chakras.html

Healing Music
www.neuroacoustic.com
www.markromeromusic.com/
www.heathernoell.com/
www.wholetones.com

HeartMath stress reduction
www.heartmath.com

Appendix B

Recommended Reading:

Chemical Sensitivities:
Explaining "Unexplained Illnesses"; by Martin L. Pall, PhD
Strategies for Surviving Chemical Sensitivities – The Basics by: Dr. Robert Mayer
Less-Toxic Alternatives; by Carolyn Gorman with Marie Hyde
Say Good-Bye to Illness; by Devi S. Nambudripad, DC

Diet:
Healing Is Voltage: by Dr. Jerry Tennant, M.D.
Eat To Live; by Joel Furhman, M.D.
The China Study; by T. Collins Campbell, PhD and Thomas M. Campbell, MD
Healthy Healing; by Linda Page, ND

EMF
Cross Currents; by Robert O. Becker, MD and Gary Selden
Dirty Electricity: by Samuel Milham, M.D., MPH
Zapped: by Anne Louise Gittleman
Electromagnetic Health: by Case Adams
Electromagnetic Sensitivity and Electromagnetic Hypersensitivity: by Michael Bevington
An Electronic Silent Spring: by Katie Singer

Energy Healing
Earthing; by Clinton Ober, Stephen Sinatra, MD, and Martin Zucker
Energy Medicine – The Scientific Basis; by James H. Oschman and Candace Pert
Healing Is Voltage 3rd Edition: by Dr. Jerry Tennant, M.D
Spring Forest Qigong; by Chunyi Lin
Tapping the Body's Energy Pathways; by Dr. Roger Callahan and Joanne Callahan

Tapping The Healer Within: by Dr. Roger Callahan
The EFT Manual – 2nd Edition; by Gary Craig
Seven Minutes to Natural Pain Release (WHEE) ; by Dr. Daniel Benor
Energy Medicine: by C. Norman Shealy, M.D.
Energy Medicine: by Donna Eden, David Feinstein, Caroline Myss

General Health
Healing Is Voltage – 3rd Edition: by Dr. Jerry Tennant, M.D.
Iodine- Why You Need It-Why You Can't Live Without It: by Dr. David Brownstein
Hypothyroidism Type 2: by Dr. Mark Starr, M.D.
Mind Over Medicine-Scientific Proof That You Can Heal Yourself: by Lissa Rankin, M. D

Inspirational:
Love, Medicine & Miracles: by Bernie Siegel, MD
The Field: the Quest for the Secret Force of the Universe, Lynne McTaggart
How Can I Heal What Hurts?: by Daniel J. Benor, MD.

Mind/Body Healing:
Biology of Belief; by Bruce H. Lipton, PhD
The HeartMath Solution; by Doc Childre and Howard Martin
Molecules Of Emotion: The Science Behind Mind-Body Medicine: by Candace Pert

Appendix C

Product Resources: *Please Note - I receive no financial benefit from any of these companies by having them listed in this book or recommending them.*

Vitamins/Nutritional Supplements:
Dr. Martin Pall's [PhD] nutritional supplementation protocol:
www.prohealth.com

Mother Earth Labs: Humic/Fulvic based nutrition
www.motherearthlabs.com

Oceans Alive Marine Phytoplankton:
www.activationproducts.com

Isotonix Vitamin B; Isotonix Digestive Enzymes, Complete Greens, and Ultimate Aloe
www.shop.com/jamazing

Crystal Energy (add to water)
www.phisciences.com

Vitamin D3 Serum from Premier Research
www.naturalhealthyconcepts.com

Detoxing
Sonne's #7 - Colloidal Bentonite
www.sonnes.com

L.L.Magnetic Clay (clay baths)
www.magneticclay.com

EMF Shielding/Protection:
Earth Calm 'whole house' EMF scalar protective device; EMF protective products for computers, mobile devices, personal wear
www.earthcalm.com

Total Shield and Personal Harmonizer from Senergy Medical Group
www.senergy.us/emf-environmental-stabilizer.html

EMF shielding products; Indoor Tent/Room; shielding for computers, cable box receivers, cell phones, televisions, etc.
www.less-emf.com

Earthing products:
www.earthing.com

General Health:
Earthing (natural grounding) products
Earthing.com

Music for Healing:
Delta, Theta Brain Wave Music
www.neuroacoustic.com

www.markromero.com
www.heathernoell.com

Non-Toxic Household cleaners:
Basic H – made by Shaklee
www.shaklee.com/shop

Stress Reduction:
HeartMath emWave program to promote heart and brain coherence
www.heartmathstore.com

Tests:
Hormonal (saliva): www.optimalhealthnetwork.com

Iodine Load Test: www.motherearthlabs.com

Appendix D

MCS, ES/EMF Sensitivity: To Do NOW List

Critical aspects are (a) the Autonomic Nervous System being out of balance -Sympathetic dominance- from one or more, usually a combination: illness, prolonged stress, injury, toxic environmental exposures, trauma, infections, etc. (b) nutritional deficiencies (c) low overall voltage (d) blockages/disturbances in the body's energy pathways.

My recommendations to a friend to consider doing immediately for EITHER MCS or EHS/EMF Sensitivity

1) Treat the condition/s with the utmost seriousness.

2) If I had MCS I would avoid not only toxic chemicals but also avoid exposure to EMF as much as possible due to how EMF spikes the same out of control NO/ONOO cycle. If I had ES/EMF sensitivity I would avoid both EMF and toxic chemicals for the same reason. These are 'sister' conditions.

3) If working, try to find a Doctor that either recognizes MCS and/or EHS or is compassionate about my circumstance for assistance as needed with medical leave, accommodations, etc. Use MCS America's Physician Referral list. If at all possible, I would take off work for a few months to avoid exposures and heal. Sacrifice right up front will be far less than it will be if these conditions get out of control.

4) Bedding/mattress: Good sleep is a valuable aid in healing

   a) In almost all cases the mattress should be covered to block chemicals, fine dust particles, etc. Organic cotton mattress protectors are all designed to breathe so my concern they still allow too much to pass through, especially gases from newer mattresses. So far food grade polyethylene looks like the best bet. It is inert. One place they can be purchased at: www.offgassing-mattress-wraps.com/ , a service from The Mom Pack : www.mompack.com/

b) Probably all cotton bedding is the best, organic cotton even better but may not be necessary. I would try washing cotton all bedding (even new organic cotton) in vinegar by first running apple cider vinegar and hot water as an empty load to clean out the washing machine, then pre- soaking the bedding for an hour or so in the washer with a 3 cups of apple cider vinegar and hot water. Some do fine even with polyester -type fill comforters that have been washed this way. It is worth the try.

c) Bed Frame: Headboard and footboards: I would remove any metal head or foot board, and any newer or freshly painted or varnished ones as well, and for sure any that are made of particle board materials where any of the particle board is exposed. That would include any side rails. Many mattresses have coil springs, and these may be a problem with EMF Sensitivity, however the Earthing mentioned next may be adequate protection to get by with the coils. Getting any replacement mattress has its own complexities, even an organic one at $2000.00 plus. It may take weeks to get, then needs to be out-gassed (yes even organic ones), so I want to make what we have work.

d) Earthing - get an Earthing pillow case, half sheet, or full mattress cover/sheet from Earthing.com and start using it immediately.

5) Minimize Chemical Exposures: Every exposure spikes the NO/ONOO cycle and makes it more difficult for or bodies to heal

a) Stop all use of all typical household cleaning products, personal care products with harmful chemicals, and non-organic lawn care products. Use vinegar and water, baking Soda for counter tops, bath tubs ,etc., and use Shaklee Basic H or similar for floors, walls, windows, and laundry.
b) Do not paint or varnish with anything but No VOC paint/varnish (no painting/varnishing best)
c) No adding new carpet or rugs to the home. I would remove any newer area rugs, or if needed for safety (like footing on a hard floor-try washing with vinegar and water or Shaklee Basic H either by hand or with a carpet cleaning machine. If you have newer carpet do the same cleaning and get as much fresh air in the home as possible if it is warm enough to do so.
d) Eliminate ALL air fresheners! in the home and car
e) Air Cleaner/Filter: With newer carpet of fresh paint or other things that may be giving off VOCs, it may be necessary to purchase an air cleaner/filter that eliminates VOCs. Otherwise, good portable room size HEPA air cleaners can be adequate. These are important to minimize dust, pollen, animal dander, mold spores, etc. to reduce your burden from these exposures. It may take two or more units to give adequate protection. I would also use a high quality furnace filter and change it regularly.
f) At work: Consider seeking accommodation for MCS or EHS/EMF Sensitivity. My understanding is that those of us having these conditions will usually be able to be covered by the Federal American with Disabilities Act (A.D.A.). http://askjan.org/media/mcs.html
g) If it was at all possible financially, I would get a portable room size air cleaner/filter unit that remove VOCs and have it right next to me. Using a small desk fan to distribute air can really be helpful whenever someone nearby is using or wearing something that causes a reaction.

6) Minimize EMF exposures: These exposures are harmful and also spike the NO/ONOO cycle just as toxic chemicals do so they need to be avoided as much as possible to heal both MCS and EMF Sensitivity.

   a) At Home: Contact your utility companies to see if you have a **Smart Meter**! Check on an Opt-Out program to get it replaced with older style meter, and/or get the Home EMF Protection Unit (Infinity) from EarthCalm company. It plugs into a wall outlet and has a number of stages of 'strength' that the user implements over a period of time. Turn off all wireless and hard-wire your internet connections if they must stay on. . Eliminate all usage or shield computers and monitor with grounded products from places like less EMF. Shield TV cable or satellite receiver unit and TV screen. Eliminate any cordless phones and replace with corded ones. Minimize use of cell phones and use a hands-free headset. Do not leave cell phone near you, especially at night. Remove all lamps, alarm clocks from nightstands. If you live in an apartment or other multi-dwelling unit, consider a device from Earth Calm that plugs into a wireless router that they claim actually protects you from the harmful effects of WiFi. Consider trying cell phone/smart phone protective devices from companies such as EarthCalm. **Note: If you are very sensitive there may not be a feeling of immediate relief form earth Calm or these steps -you need to do all essentials for a while and need to down regulate the NO/ONOO Cycle.**

   b) If you live with others and cannot do most of these things, consider products from EarthCalm We use the EarthCalm Whole House Protection device and feel it is an life saver and allowed my wife to get well over time. Consider their personal protection devices.

c) Earthing while on a computer or near a TV and receiver will also offer protection from EMF. Using wrist bands or special Earthing pads from Earthing.com. This is a good way to get protection at work if we have to keep working through your healing time, as well as at home when we absolutely need to use a computer there.

d) ***For ultimate and immediate protection from EMF at home, get the indoor tent/room called the Quiet Zone Retreat for about $500 from lessEMF.com!***

7) Supplements

Comprehensive Wellness (humic/fulvic base) or pH Balancer from Mother Earth Labs: I would start out with 1/3 or 1/2 the normal dose for a few weeks then gradually increase it to a normal or even above normal dosage (2-3 ounces) during healing. In brief, this one product may cover the vast majority of our nutritional needs an in the form our body's cells can readily utilize, dramatically improve PH, removes toxins including mercury and other heavy metals very effectively, even from deep inside our cells and safely, and more. Extensive information is available at motherearthlabs.com. Have someone download the free booklet and print it out for detailed info and excellent suggestions for health and healing. Alkalizing Diet information is also provided in the booklet.

B Vitamin complex- helps balance the Autonomic Nervous System-a key to healing these conditions. We prefer Isotonix Activated B Complex from Market America.

Oceans Alive Marine Phytoplankton for another complete, readily absorbed whole food source of a broad array of minerals, amino acids, essential fatty acids, and vitamins. Plus, it is an excellent source of high quality, bioavailable of the powerful anti-oxidant

SOD (Superoxide Dismutase) – ***this alone might stop the vicious NO/ONOO Cycle!***

Lugol's Plus Iodine (Iodine/Potassium Iodide with needed cofactors) supplement from Mother Earth Labs: Almost everyone in western cultures is very short of Iodine and it is very critical for good health. If any doubts about needing it, we would get the **Iodine Load Test** from Mother Earth Labs to confirm if I was low.

Vitamin D3: Too important to be short of and most of us are very low. I like 5,000 IU/day for a maintenance level. If I had blood work that showed I was really low, I would take up to 10,000 IU/day for a month or two. A quality D3 from a natural source is important.

8) Foods and Water

Green Drink: Find a good quality one that you like and will use.

Some general guidelines: Avoid processed foods. Lean towards an alkalizing diet. Organic fruits and vegetables are best-eat half as much if needed due to the expense. Use mostly organic whole grains. Avoid soy products. Get adequate essential fatty acids from organic flaxseed oil, chai seeds, coconut oil, organic butter, and high quality purified fish or krill oils. Avoid canola oil, caffeine, artificial sweeteners.

Whey protein (non-denatured) is not only a great source for protein but provides the body what it needs to make its own glutathione (best way to get it) -the Master Antioxidant and the Director of Detoxification.

Drink sufficient amounts of pure water: Reverse Osmosis is a good option without using expensive home filtration units. Adding Crystal Energy [www.phisciences.com] is a good option.

9) Balance the Autonomic Nervous System (ANS)

   a) The EarthCalm Whole House Unit or the Total Shield, B Vitamins, and Earthing device are all very helpful for balancing the ANS

   b) Use TFT-Thought Field Therapy meridian tapping several times a day for a while. This has a quick and dramatic positive effect on balancing the Autonomic Nervous System. Download one of the free guides for Stress or Trauma generously offered at: http://tfttraumarelief.com/instructions-for-tft-trauma-relief-technique/

   c) Correct "Bowling Ball Syndrome". Dr. Jerry Tenant, M D finds that almost everyone with chronic illness has this condition and it greatly impedes healing. The best health can come when the ANS (Autonomic Nervous System) is in balance, as the Parasympathetic is responsible for most healing activities and cannot function correctly if the Sympathetic is dominant.

   To see if we are 'Sympathetic stuck in on mode", look straight ahead and have someone see if one ear lobe is lower (even slightly) than the other and one shoulder (same or opposite side) is slightly lower than the other. If so then we have this condition. Another indicator is to stand still, looking straight ahead and if you are still and do not slightly sway back and forth about 10 times per minute, and if not, then the Sympathetic nervous system is stuck on.

   To correct this use Life Wave 'Energy' patches [lifewave.com], applying one on each side of the neck (White patch on right side and Tan patch on left side) on the 'Autonomic Reset' point on the right side of the neck and the same location on the left side . This spot is a little beyond half way down the distance between bottom of ear lobe and shoulder, and centered on a line straight down from the outer edge of ear] See drawings. Leave on about 6-8 hours and recheck ear lobes. If they are level, recheck them periodically (shoulders take 24 hours to level out). If not, leave patches on longer or do again another day, then recheck. Check also by standing still and seeing if your body now sways back and forth slightly about 10 times per minute. This will indicate the condition has been corrected. Keep checking every few days and re-apply if needed to keep level. Dr. Tennant finds that low overall body voltage is the main reason the correction does not hold. Earthing 6-8 hours and Mother Earth labs Comprehensive Wellness should improve and maintain overall body voltage.

10) Promote internal energetic calmness

    a) Highly recommended for immediate relief! Use the "Un-Switching Protocol" from Deena Zalkind Spear, a one minute exercise that helps 'unscramble' crossed electrical signals that are a result of chemical, physical, environmental, nutritional or emotional stresses. I would be sure to use it several times a day. I believe that by getting our internal energies in greater harmony we are more naturally shielded from EMF. A free download of the protocol is generously offered by Deena at www.singingwoods.org. Try it and you will know it is helping.

    b) Use Bach's Rescue Remedy flower essence throughout the day, every 20-30 minutes or so if needed. Can add to water and sip it.

    c) Deep Breathing Technique: place had on belly, breathe in slowly for count of 7, feeling belly expand; hold for count of 5; breathe out through mouth for count of 5. Repeat for several minutes.

ABOUT THE AUTHOR

This is Gary's first book. It came to be as a result of searching relentlessly for a remedy/cure for his wife's extreme chemical and EMF sensitivities.

Natural healing modalities and their application to disease became a passion for Gary when his father was diagnosed with cancer and proved an invaluable healing influence with his own 4th stage cancer diagnosis ten years later.

Gary lives with his lovely wife of 41 years, is the proud father of two fine sons and a grandfather of the light of his life, his granddaughter.

CPSIA information can be obtained
at www.ICGtesting.com
Printed in the USA
BVHW03s0217170418
513596BV00018B/271/P